Human
COMMUNICATION

Human
COMMUNICATION
A Linguistic Introduction

Graham Williamson

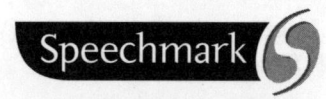
Speechmark ⑤

Speechmark Publishing Ltd
Telford Road, Bicester, Oxon OX26 4LQ, UK

Graham Williamson is a speech & language therapist with experience of the NHS, private sector and independent practice. He has worked extensively with people with learning disabilities. In 1990 he received a Master's degree in Research Methods from the Open University, and in 1995 a PhD from Newcastle University, having studied conversation analysis. His interest is the popularisation of human communication issues among non-specialists.

First published in 2001 by
Speechmark Publishing Ltd, Telford Road, Bicester, Oxon OX26 4LQ, United Kingdom
www.speechmark.net

© Graham Williamson, 2001
www.grahamwilliamson.com

002-4215/Printed in the United Kingdom/1010

British Library Cataloguing in Publication Data

Williamson, Graham
   Human communication: a linguistic introduction. – (Winslow editions)
   1. Oral communication   2. Sociolinguistics
   I. Title
   302.2'24
ISBN 0 86388 236 6

For Margaret, Daniel, Adam and Kathryn Mary

Contents

Figures

Tables

Foreword

THE ABILITY TO COMMUNICATE is a feature of many forms of life. However, the use of complex and flexible spoken language is unique to human beings. Furthermore, humans have the ability to communicate about their communication in different ways. They have a language with which to talk about language or write about language. This 'metalinguistic awareness', as it is called, means that they are able to analyse language and discuss ways in which one language differs from another, or one person's communication skills differ from those of another person. They can manipulate and explore language, using it in different ways for different purposes. Human beings can talk about language from the perspectives of its meaning, its structure and its function. This introduction to human communication exploits the unique human facility to discuss language and communication. In doing so, the book provides an opportunity for people with an interest in human communication to learn about language and understand how it works. The ability to talk is often taken for granted. Children usually learn to do this without having to be taught directly. By the time they start school, children have largely mastered the complex skills of putting sounds together to make words, and words together to make meaningful utterances. It is assumed that teachers will teach and children will learn through language, and that language will provide a foundation for all of our relationships with each other.

This book focuses on human communication from a linguistic perspective, looking at how it works and how it varies. People in all walks of life are likely to find the insights useful. The general reader and friends and family members of people with communication difficulties will find it helpful to understand more of the detail underlying communication skills; teachers and others in caring roles will benefit from insight into the ways in which communication can vary; students of language will find the presentation of linguistic concepts, together with the revision exercises and activities, particularly useful. In summary, this book is about a normal human activity, talking, which is surely of interest to most of us.

Carol Miller
School of Education, University of Birmingham

Preface

THIS BOOK INVESTIGATES *COMMUNICATION*. The word is familiar, but it is likely that we each have a different idea of exactly what it means. It appears within the common vernacular in various forms:

she's a good *communicator*
communication is the key to a successful marriage
Captain Kirk *communicated* with the alien

Ordinarily, we do not think about how we communicate: it is taken for granted that we organise and live our lives through this process. In reality, it is one of the most important activities in which human beings engage. This book is designed to help you think more carefully about the process of communication. But not just any kind of communication. The emphasis here is on *human* communication and not, for example, animal communication. While animal communication is an extremely interesting area of study, this book does not explore it in any depth. A few examples of the differences between animal and human communication are provided, but the primary focus remains human communication. There are many approaches to the study and each is informed by a different discipline. There are philosophical approaches, psychological, biological, and so on. In this book, however, we will take a distinctively linguistic approach. Loosely speaking, linguistics may be defined as the scientific study of language. However, this definition may suggest that speech, as a facet of human communication, is not incorporated under the rubric of linguistics. For our purposes, therefore, we will assume a general definition of linguistics that subsumes these two major aspects of human communication – language and speech. We will adopt the concepts and categories of the field of general linguistics. This approach to the study of human communication is typically concerned with examining such things as the structure and function of language, the ways in which language is acquired, the physiological mechanisms for speech production, and the interdependence of language and culture. Clearly, the field is vast and in this introductory book we can only provide an overview of some of these major areas. Generally, the selected topics will be exemplified by reference to normal development. In other words, we will set out the main themes in relation to how one might expect a normally developing person to acquire and use specific communication skills. This is not a book about pathology – ie, what can go wrong in the development of human communication. However, occasional reference to disorders will be made where these are capable of contrasting and highlighting important areas of normal human communication. A final point is that the particular world language that forms the focus of this book is English. English is the fourth most common language spoken throughout the world, being spoken by about 1,000 million people. The most common language is Mandarin Chinese, then Hindi, Spanish and English. There are, of course, many variants of English: American English, Australian English, and so on. In most instances, and especially when commenting on the pronunciation of speech sounds, we will be referring to southern British English throughout.

As an introductory text, this book is aimed at non-specialists who have an interest – professional or otherwise – in understanding more of the process of human communication. It is suitable for both the general reader, and for people wishing to explore this particular field. It will also be a useful resource for professionals wishing to pass on ideas on human communication through talks, presentations and workshops. In addition, it should prove useful to those interested in teaching English as a foreign language (TEFL).

Outline

The book is divided into four main parts: (1) the nature of human communication, (2) language, (3) speech, and (4) conversation. The first part sets the scene and presents a context for later discussions. There is a logical progression as far as the presentation of the remaining parts goes – ie, language → speech → conversation – in that conversation presupposes competency in both speech and language, and the ability to communicate effectively through speech presupposes the possession of language. Each chapter ends with revision exercises that test your understanding of the material in the chapter and activities that help consolidate learning. A key to the exercises is provided towards the end of the book.

Part 1: The Nature of Human Communication

The first part, consisting of Chapter 1, explores the general nature of human communication and begins by constructing a working definition. The concepts of language, speech and non-verbal communication are then introduced. In broad terms, language is the ability to understand and use symbols (words); speech is the transmission system of language, and non-verbal communication refers to the variety of ways in which human beings transmit meaning to one another other than by spoken language. Subsequently, a set of prerequisite skills for developing human communication is considered, before a model of human communication known as the *Communication Chain* is introduced. This model is useful as a visual representation of the process of human communication. It can be referred to throughout your reading in order to set the various topics of discussion into the context of the whole process of human communication. The chapter concludes with a brief look at conversation – the archetypal language use through which people participate in social interactions.

Part 2: Language

The second part focuses on language and consists of Chapters 2 to 5.

Language properties, acquisition and development
Chapter 2 begins by noting that language is the predominant means by

which human beings communicate with each other. It then outlines eight key properties of language that help to explain why this is so. The difficult issue of how language is acquired by children is then addressed by means of considering four possible explanations: probability, imitation, cognition, and a genetically pre-programmed innate ability. While discussing the last of these explanations, we consider briefly animal communication. Focusing primarily on ape research, we consider whether or not these primates are able to demonstrate any of the key properties of language that are an invariant feature of human language. The chapter then concludes with an overview of the development of language from the so-called pre-linguistic stage through to the production of complex linguistic utterances at around 48–60 months of age.

Building and combining words
Chapters 3 and 4 take up the theme of expressive language – ie, how words are formed and subsequently sequenced to create meaningful utterances. Chapter 3 provides a description of morphology and considers how such things as prefixes and suffixes can be added to single words in order to create new words and, therefore, new meanings. We also introduce the nine word classes of English: nouns, verbs, adjectives, adverbs, numerals, determiners, pronouns, prepositions and conjunctions. Each class is explained in turn. Chapter 4 moves on to consider not simply words in isolation, but how several words can combine to create phrases, which in turn combine to form clauses. This area of study is known as syntax. Syntax explores the rules that define which particular word types can be combined legitimately and the rules governing the correct sequencing of these words.

Language meaning and language use
Humans are social beings and we spend a great deal of our time functioning in communities with other people. We know that different social groups attach different meanings to particular behaviours and ways of doing things. The use of language is a specific behaviour and various meanings may be attached to how people use language in particular social settings. Chapter 5 explores some of the social dimensions of language use. We consider first how meaning is attributed to words and phrases.

This is the study of semantics. Next we consider the social use of language – eg, how a person may make an active choice to speak in a certain style to one person and yet choose a completely different style when speaking to another person. This is the domain of pragmatics.

Part 3: Speech
The third part of the book considers the second major aspect of human communication: speech. This part is covered by Chapters 6 to 8.

Speech sounds
As we have seen, speech is the transmission system of language. It involves rapid, coordinated movements of the lips, tongue, palate of the mouth, vocal folds and breathing to articulate sounds that are used to form meaningful words. In English there is a fixed number of speech sounds and these are divided into two categories: vowels and consonants. Following some definitions of speech, Chapter 6 provides a description of the articulation of both types of speech sound. The pronunciation of particular speech sounds is not always constant, however, and their pronunciation may vary according to the context in which they occur. These variations are known as allophones and they are discussed towards the end of the chapter. The study of how speech sounds are articulated is known as phonetics.

The speech sound system
Phonology refers to the rule system governing the permitted sound combinations in any language. Phonology is introduced in Chapter 7, and the organisation of speech sounds at three different levels – phonemic, syllabic and word – is described. The majority of the chapter, however, is devoted to an examination of the various ways in which words may be reformulated through an alteration to their basic structure or through other systematic changes, such as the substitution of one speech sound for another.

Connected speech
It is self-evident that humans do not generally speak one word at a time. Rather, we converse with each other by producing sequences of words in

a continuous stream known as connected speech. Chapter 8 begins by considering the factors that influence the movement of the articulatory mechanism when producing connected speech in real time. We then see how the pronunciation of words may alter in rapidly delivered connected speech, and we examine a number of systematic processes that operate at the boundary between one word and another. Connected speech also has a characteristic rhythmical beat and an attendant musical quality. This is known as prosody and it is examined next. Finally, the chapter concludes with a consideration of factors that may influence the production of smooth, uninterrupted and fluent speech.

Part 4: Conversation

Part 4 of the book consists solely of Chapter 9. In this part we examine conversation in relation to its overall management, and especially how turns at talk are allocated in real time. First we set out some of the chief characteristics of conversation, then we present a fundamental unit of conversation known as an adjacency pair. Next we explore how turns at talk are allocated in conversations and introduce a set of rules that govern this process. The highly collaborative nature of conversation is seen to be operative through the application of these rules and we reflect on the fact that participants in a conversation generally talk one at a time. Next we examine instances when this general tendency to talk one at a time is infringed. This is the phenomenon of overlapping talk, and we investigate why certain overlaps are considered to be accidental and yet others are thought to be wilful interruptions. The chapter closes with a brief look at how conversational participants resolve the conflict of overlapping talk.

For further information and articles on speech and language issues see the website **www.grahamwilliamson.com**.

Graham Williamson
November 2000

Acknowledgements

THIS BOOK EMERGED over a number of years in the course of working as a speech and language therapist for South Durham Health Care NHS Trust and as a Regional Tutor for the School of Education, University of Birmingham. I have long been interested in promoting an understanding of the theoretical underpinnings of human communication as a means to working with people who present with disorders of communication. My work has led me to design several courses aimed at assisting people with little or no knowledge of the field to understand this extraordinarily fascinating topic. It has brought me into direct contact with a wide range of professional and lay people, including teachers, non-teaching staff, occupational therapists, physiotherapists, clinical and educational psychologists, speech & language therapists and assistants, and students. I therefore wish to extend my gratitude to all those whom I have had the privilege to teach, especially for their constructive feedback on the materials and methods used, much of which has found its way into this book. My students at the University of Birmingham continue to be a source of challenge and motivation and their contribution is inestimable. I would also like to thank Stephanie Martin at Winslow Press for her helpful comments on an earlier draft and to Carol Miller at the University of Birmingham for her Foreword. Finally, I extend my heartfelt thanks to my immediate family who, as always, have lovingly supported me, and it is to them that I dedicate this book.

CHAPTER 1

The Nature of Human Communication

THE GENTLE TOUCH of someone's hand. Numbers on a computer screen. Picasso's *Guernica*. The music of the great, and not so great, composers. A romantic novel. The persuasive oration of a government official. The cry of a small child. All these are commonly held to be acts of communication. Take music, for example. Music may excite an emotion, arouse a mood or convey an impression of energy. Similarly, a painting may awaken consciousness and a sense of the artist's purpose. Such art forms have the power to call forth feelings of intimacy and romance or of terror and foreboding. Mathematics, however, tends not to invoke mood, humour or the vagaries of human disposition. It is more grounded in laws, rules and solutions. Consider touch. The soft, gentle caress of love clearly communicates an entirely different message from the hard, brutal slap of aggression. We talk of those who communicate confidence and of some as being good communicators. The implication is that there are people who are bad at communicating. This suggests an underlying presumption that communication is a skill. And if it is a skill then, surely, it can be taught and learnt? We talk of the intensity of the information transmitted in an act of communication: 'It was a powerful message'. And of the intensity of the medium: 'It was a powerful painting'. And of the intensity of the communicator: 'She is a powerful speaker'. But does the witty, playful discourse of an experienced public speaker engage one's attention and communicate any more forcefully than the cry of a distressed child?

Paintings are one means of representing the appearance of the world. Music is another. Maths is another, and so on. We may not, though, consider ourselves to be artists, musicians or mathematicians. Indeed, we may have no experience of attempting to communicate by these means. However, most of us will have direct experience of accomplishing communication by the use of words. As we shall see, it is human capacity to build words, combine these into meaningful sequences and then articulate them through speech that makes them the most powerful communicators on the planet. The verbal aspect of communication is the major focus of this book. We will begin our investigation of this fascinating area of study by attempting to construct a working definition of human communication.

What is Human Communication?

As noted in the Preface, this book seeks to investigate communication and, specifically, human communication. In this section we will construct a working definition of human communication.

Communication Situations

Consider the number of different situations in which you had to communicate yesterday. Spend a few moments now to jot down some ideas below.

Situations in which I communicated yesterday

The number and types of situations in which we communicate are virtually limitless. Clearly your list will reflect who you are, what sort of activities you enjoy, whether you are in formal employment, and so on. Your list of situations may include some of the following: asking for a bus ticket; explaining to an employer why you have not completed an assignment; ordering lunch; singing in a choir; shouting at a child! Evidently we all spend a great deal of our time communicating with others. In fact, human beings have been described as 'compulsive communicators'. But what do all these examples of communication have in common? Imagine for a moment that you were visiting a friend whom you had not seen for some time. The chances are that you would spend a lot of time talking to each other. You would probably ask your friend several questions to find out what they had been doing since the last time you met, how they felt about living where they do, what the latest gossip was, and so on. It is likely that your friend would answer most, if not all, of your questions and would probably ask you a few as well. By the time you left you would have gathered a great deal of information from your friend, and also given them a good deal of information in exchange. This purposeful act of passing messages from one speaker to another is a fairly typical aspect of what might be described as human communication. But must all communication merely involve the passing of messages?

Reasons for Communicating
While messages such as, 'I saw *Les Miserables* last night,' 'I want a return ticket to Newcastle,' and 'Duncan is an instrument artificer' clearly involve some sort of informing, the previous example of singing in a choir does not appear to involve sending the same type of message. Is telling someone that I have been to the theatre the same type of message as informing a close friend that I have a terminal illness? There would appear to be many different reasons for communicating. Take a few more moments to list below some of the possible reasons why humans might choose to communicate with others.

Reasons for communicating
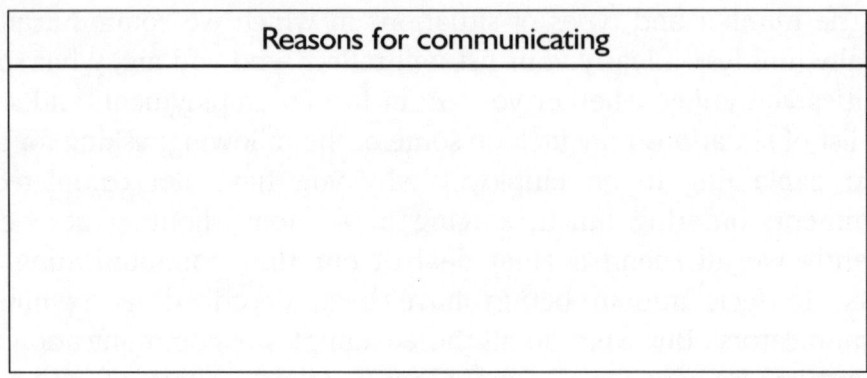

Again, the number seems almost limitless. Some examples include: transmitting ideas; sharing information; passing messages; telling stories to make someone laugh; calming down an anxious person; expressing love; declaring an allegiance; teaching a skill; asking questions; threatening someone; expressing emotion, and persuading.

Intention, Agency and Recipiency

Considering the types of situations in which we communicate and the reasons for doing so, it appears that communication involves at least three things: (1) intention, (2) agency, and (3) recipiency. That is to say, someone (the agent) intentionally instigates a communicative behaviour, eg, they speak a message. However, on its own, this act is insufficient to be described as communicative. An act is only communicative if it is subsequently received by another person (the recipient). Typically, communicative acts, as we have seen, are aimed at instituting some change in the recipient. For example, if I inform a stranger where I live then I intend to bring about a change in the stranger's knowledge, and if I ask a child to be quiet I intend to change the child's noisiness. In summary:

Communication is an intentional act performed by an agent for the purpose of causing some effect in a recipient.

Non-Human Agents

In the examples cited so far all the agents are human beings. Suppose, however, that a dog places its foot in its empty water bowl and barks.

Subsequent to this its human owner picks up the bowl, fills it with water and returns it to the dog, which then drinks the water. Has communication taken place? Well, according to our summary definition, we would have to conclude that it has. Agents, of course, do not just have to be human beings. They can be any animate being which is capable of acting with intent. In the situation just described this would include the dog. The dog has intentionally transmitted a signal to a recipient (its owner) and it has created an effect in this recipient (ie, the owner went and filled its water bowl). Similarly, recipients can also be non-human, as when a human owner (agent) instructs the dog (recipient) to, 'Sit!' The primary purpose of this book is not to consider communication which is instigated by non-human agents or which is intended for receipt by non-human recipients. In other words, we are concerned solely with human communication. Our summary definition should, therefore, be amended to read:

Human communication is an intentional act performed by a human agent for the purpose of causing some effect in a human recipient.

Language

There are important differences between animal communication and human communication. Some of these relate to the fact that only human beings appear to be genetically pre-programmed to learn what is known as language. Language is the predominant means by which human beings communicate with each other. In broad terms, language is an ability to understand and use symbols. Humans especially make use of verbal symbols (ie, the spoken word) for thinking and communicating. Several researchers have attempted to teach language skills to animals, most notably apes (see, for example, Gardner & Gardner, 1969; Premack, 1970, 1971; Terrace, 1979; Savage-Rumbaugh & Lewin, 1994). However, animals do not appear to have an innate predisposition for learning language. While they may be taught the rudiments of a language, they typically do not progress beyond the ability level of a 2;06[1] year-old human child. In addition, humans are able to use language to describe novel events and situations which have happened in the past, and which will happen in the future. Moreover, we can communicate concrete ideas about the here-and-now as well as abstract concepts such as feelings, attitudes and perceptions. There is seemingly a near-infinite flexibility to what human beings are capable of communicating. In comparison, while the dances of bees may be considered to be a form of communication, it is extremely limited. Their dances are capable of communicating the specific location of a food source but they could not, for example, describe how hot it was the day before yesterday or what they intend to do tomorrow. In stark contrast, any normally developed human being would have no difficulty communicating these concepts, and it is language that enables them to do so. Two facets of language are usually described. The first is receptive language or comprehension, which involves our ability to understand the verbal symbols spoken to us. The second is expressive language, which comprises our ability to produce meaningful utterances through an appropriate use of vocabulary, word order and such things as word endings. Any particular language, such as English, French or Hindi, is governed by a discrete set of rules known as the grammar of the language. The grammatical rules specify, for example, which words (symbols) can be combined with which others, what constitutes a meaningful word, and so on. Each particular language, therefore, has its own particular grammatical rules. There are, in fact, two aspects of grammar. These are known as morphology and syntax. Morphology considers the form and structure of the words used in a particular language. It examines how prefixes and suffixes can be added to a word root in order to alter its meaning. So, for example, a word root such as *heat* can be extended by adding the prefix *re-* to create the new word-meaning *reheat*. Similarly, the suffix *-ed* can be appended to create the new word-meaning *heated*. Morphology is discussed in greater depth in Chapter 3. Syntax investigates the ways in which words are related to construct meaningful utterances. Not all combinations of words are considered to be grammatically correct. So, for example, in English *the funny boy* is considered acceptable whereas *the boy funny* is not. A fuller explanation of syntax is given in Chapter 4.

Speech

Take a moment to review your list of situations in which you communicated yesterday. How many of these situations involved your having to talk to one or more people? It would not be surprising to find that a high percentage of your examples involved this behaviour. This is because, for a variety of reasons, some of which will become clear as you work through this book, human beings use speech as the most effective and flexible means of communicating ideas and sharing experiences and knowledge. This is true of all human social groups. In fact, throughout history there have been societies that have existed without being able to read or write, but we are not aware of any that have existed and did not use speech. Speech is the primary transmission system of language. It is highly complex and it has to be learnt. It involves rapid, coordinated movements of the lips, tongue, palate of the mouth, vocal folds (popularly, although inaccurately, also known as vocal cords) and breathing to articulate sounds which are then used to form meaningful words. In English there is a fixed number of speech sounds which are divided into two categories: vowels and consonants. As with language, speech has its own set of rules that govern which particular sound combinations may or may not be produced. For example, in English, the sound 'ng' is allowable at the ends of words, such as in wing, sing and ring. However, this sound never occurs at the beginning of words – ie, there are no words in English that begin with 'ng'. Phonetics is the aspect of speech that describes how the sounds are articulated through the coordinated use of the lips, tongue, teeth, palate and breath. Phonology refers to the rule system governing the permitted sound combinations in any language.

Non-Verbal Communication

While we overwhelmingly control our environment by language through the medium of speech, there are other means of communication. Consider the following:

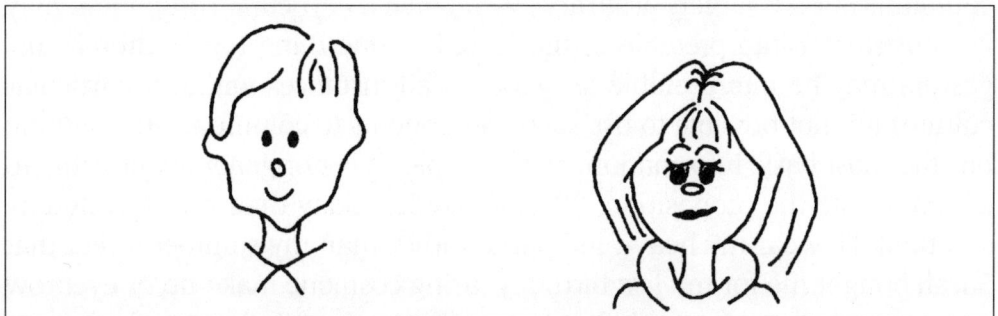

How can these two communicate if they can't speak?

How did you do? Some possible means include the following:

- writing (on paper, cloth, wax tablets, a computer screen)
- semaphore
- beating a drum
- Morse code
- smoke signals
- sign language (as used by people with hearing impairment)
- natural gestures
- body posture
- facial expression
- touch
- cosmetic make-up

While it is unlikely that you will communicate by smoke signals or semaphore it is, of course, likely that you will make use of such things as facial expression, natural gesture and body posture. These are examples of non-verbal communication and they are particularly useful when we communicate in face-to-face situations. They are helpful in enhancing our verbal communication by signalling such things as our attention, whether we are bored, whether we intend to interrupt, and so on. It is evident that some sort of meaning may be conveyed by the use of non-verbal components. However, the nature of such non-verbal communication cannot approach the exactness and creativity of verbal communication – ie, the use of spoken language. We have already touched on the reason for this limitation, which is that language is systematic whereas non-verbal communication is largely arbitrary. Even when a particular component may be consistently interpretable as meaning just one thing (eg, a 'thumbs up' gesture may be interpretable as 'good' in all instances within a particular culture) it is not possible to use such components to communicate anything but the most basic information. For example, it is not generally possible to communicate the proposition, 'It's a lot colder today than it was yesterday so I think I'll wear my heavy, red parka rather than my summer jacket that Sarah bought me for my last birthday' using cosmetic make-up or eyebrow movements! To achieve this level of sophistication we have to look once more towards a systematic use of symbols and a system that allows these symbols to be combined according to set rules. Perhaps the most obvious example of such a non-verbal communication system is manual signing, eg, British Sign Language, as used by people with hearing impairments. In a manual signing system the symbols are not words, as in spoken language, but hand shapes. Signing systems typically have their own rules, or grammar, that dictate how the various hand shapes may be combined to convey meaning. These grammars may or may not be the same as the grammar of the spoken language. However, because signing is systematic it is capable of conveying a richness of meaning that cannot be achieved through the use of other non-verbal communication components.

Prerequisites for Developing Human Communication

Many faculties and skills are necessary to become an effective communicator. These may best be considered in terms of the skills required to develop language and those that are necessary to develop speech.

Prerequisites for Language Development

1   *Cause and effect.* The developing child must realise that their actions influence other people: eg, if the child cries or lifts an arm then somebody responds. The development of this skill takes place between about 0 and 2;00 years of age. The child gradually begins to learn that it is discrete and separate from the various objects and people in its environment and begins to understand that its own actions can influence objects and people around it.

2   *Reciprocity.* The child must realise that communication is reciprocal, ie, particular behaviours on the part of other people require a response from the child. For example, if the child's mother smiles then the child could smile back.

3   *Symbolic understanding.* The symbols used in language are words and the developing child must, therefore, learn to represent objects and things in their environment by words. There is a symbol continuum that progresses from the conceptually simple to the conceptually complex (see Figure 1.1), and as the complexity of the symbols increases, so the ability to understand that one thing stands for another becomes more and more important. Between the ages of 2;00 and 7;00 years the child's vocabulary expands rapidly as they learn to represent objects by words.

4   *Memory.* Memory is the process of storing and retrieving information in the brain. It is important in learning, thinking and acquiring language. Auditory memory is particularly important, as speech is transient. What we mean by this is that when a word, or string of words, is spoken, it is heard once and then the sound disappears. The sounds do not remain for us to listen to them again in order to check our understanding or otherwise revise them. This is in contrast to the same word, or string of words, being written down. When they are written down, a permanent record is made of the message and it can be read and reread at leisure. Thus, the child needs to be able to store the auditory signal in the brain long enough to be able to process its meaning and respond appropriately.

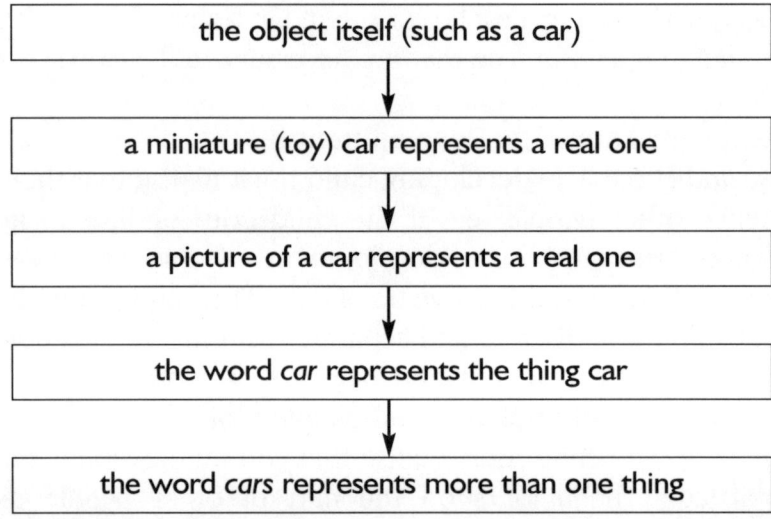

Figure 1.1 *Symbol Continuum*

Prerequisites for Speech Development

1   *Sounds.* Children must be able to make a range of different sounds and be able to make their voices rise and fall rhythmically. Specifically, a child must be physically able to produce speech sounds. These are the vowels and consonants that make up the words of the particular language that they are exposed to and, therefore, that they will speak as they grow.

2   *Hearing and listening.* Children need to be able to hear and locate sounds and they must be able to attend (listen) to those that are important and ignore those that are not. So, for example, if a child is playing with its father who is singing a nursery rhyme, there may also be a lot of background noise in the room. The background noise may include such things as the noise of a fridge humming, a bird singing outside the window or music playing. The developing child must learn to discriminate between sounds that are 'speech' sounds and those that are not.

3   *Imitation.* Children need to be able to copy a variety of speech sounds and sound patterns.

4   *Motivation.* Children must want to communicate by speech, if they are to do so successfully.

One final but important point is that a child may be physically able to produce speech sounds but may not be able to use them meaningfully unless they have understanding. In other words, the child must first have developed certain language skills that inform them how the speech sounds can be used to form meaningful words and phrases. If the sounds are used only to create random combinations then they cannot convey any substantive meaning. It is only when speech sounds are used systematically that people can be said to be communicating effectively.

The Communication Chain

How children develop the realisations and symbolic skills described in the previous section is a matter of considerable debate. We will reflect on some possible explanations in the next chapter, where we consider theories of language acquisition. For now, we will consider a model of human communication known as the *Communication Chain*. A model is merely a map that helps us to understand better particular features of a process, in this case human communication. It is, of course, not the process itself but merely a representation of it. No model can incorporate every aspect of the process it seeks to explain. However, the Communication Chain is sufficiently robust to provide a useful framework in which we can set the future topics of discussion. Figure 1.2 illustrates

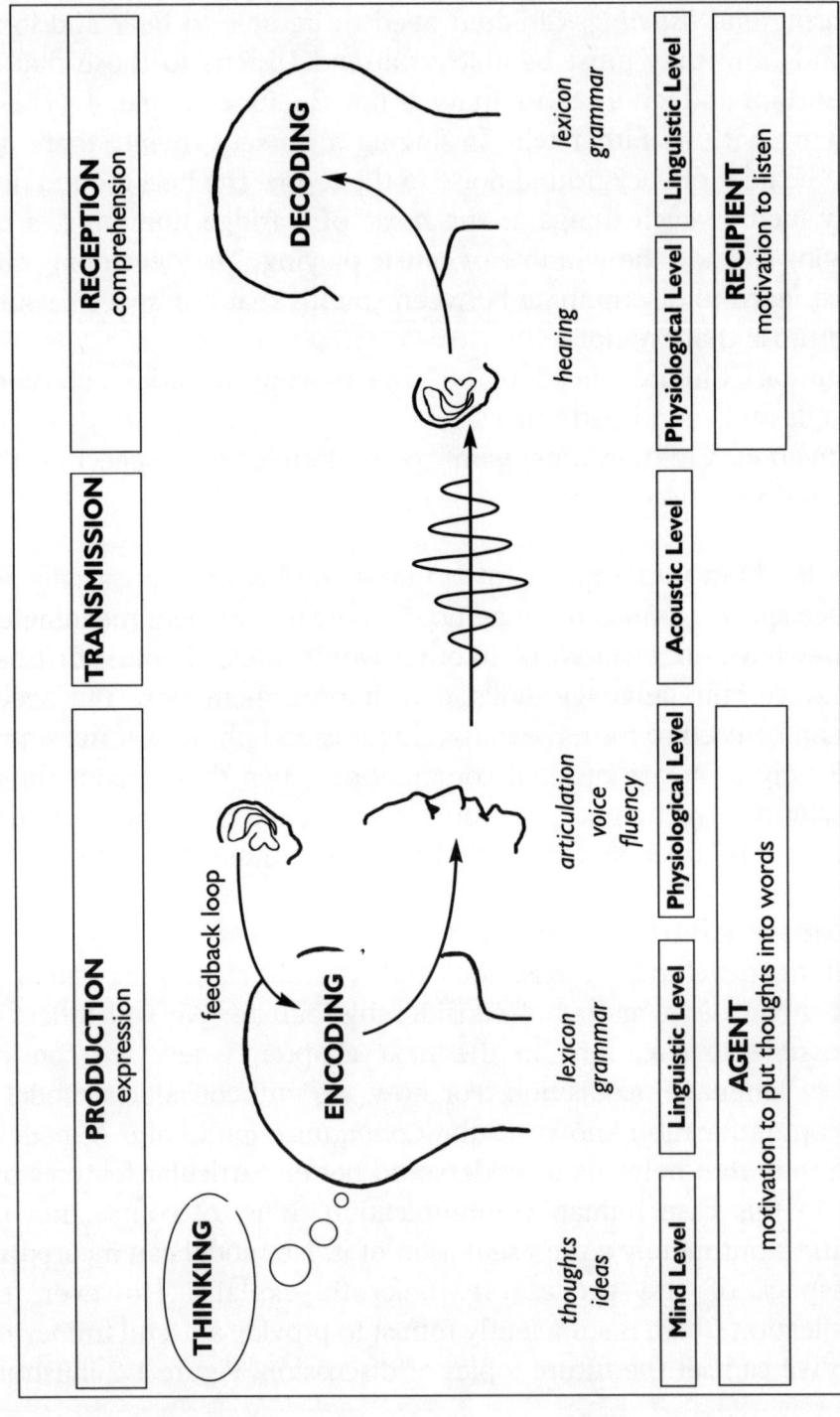

Figure 1.2 *The Communication Chain*

the Communication Chain and the following discussion, which explains the model, refers to this diagram throughout. (The model of the Communication Chain as presented here is an extension of an earlier model known as the *Speech Chain*, originally outlined by Denes and Pinson [1973; but see also their updated discussion in Denes & Pinson, 1993]; see also chapter 3 in Crystal & Varley, 1998.)

The first thing of note in Figure 1.2 is that there are three main 'links' in the Communication Chain: (1) production, (2) transmission and (3) reception.

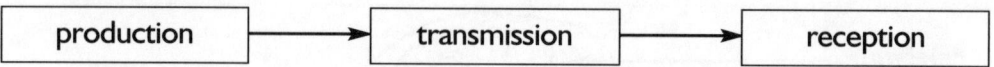

As we will see, production refers to the process by which a human agent expresses themselves by first deciding what message they wish to communicate, then planning and encoding the appropriate linguistic utterance and, finally, producing this utterance through the suitable coordination of the vocal apparatus. Production of a verbal utterance, therefore, takes place at three levels: mind, linguistic and physiological. Production is sometimes simply referred to as expression. Transmission refers to the sending of the linguistic utterance through some medium to the recipient. As we are concerned only with verbal communication in this book, there is only one medium of consequence and that is air – ie, the spoken utterance travels through the medium of air to the recipient's ear. We have already noted, when considering non-verbal communication, that there are other media through which a message could be transmitted. For example, if we were interested in a discussion of written messages then a likely medium of transmission would be ink and paper. Because we are concerned with the transmission of messages that use a so-called vocal-auditory channel, then transmission is said to occur at the acoustic level. Reception refers to the process by which the recipient of a verbal utterance detects the utterance through the sense of hearing and then decodes the linguistic expression. Reception can also be seen as operating at the two linguistic and physiological levels. Reception is often referred to as comprehension.

Mind Level

When two people talk together, the speaker (agent) sends messages to the listener (recipient) in the form of words. The speaker has first to decide what they want to say and then to choose the right words to put together in order to send the message. We do not fully understand how people think, collect their thoughts and then decide what they want to say. What we do know, however, is that these decisions are taken in a part of the brain known as the cortex. There are three major parts to the brain: (1) the cerebrum, (2) the cerebellum and (3) the brain stem (see Figure 1.3).

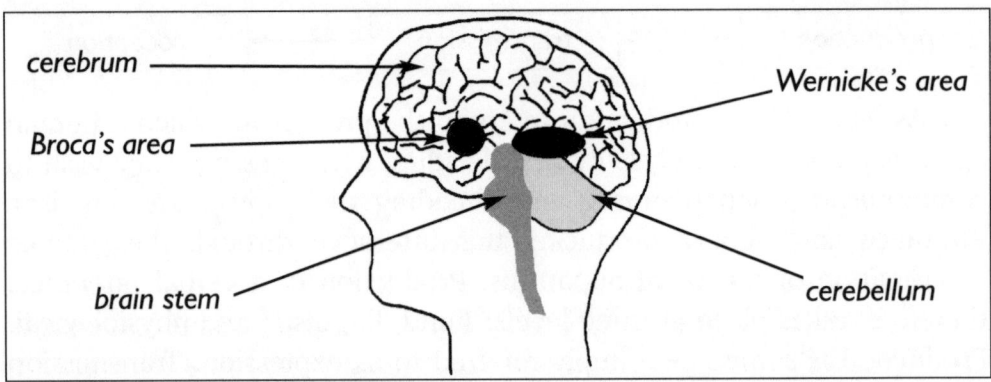

Figure 1.3 *Anatomy of the Brain*

Cerebrum

The cerebrum is divided along the longitudinal fissure into two almost identical halves: the left and the right cerebral hemispheres. The outer layer of each hemisphere is known as the cerebral cortex; it is highly convoluted, with many intricate folds. These serve to increase the surface area of the brain. The left hemisphere controls the movements of the right-hand side of the body and the right hemisphere controls the left side. In most people one of the hemispheres is dominant over the other and, for most people, it is the left hemisphere that is dominant. Therefore, most people are right-handed, as it is the left hemisphere that dominates. In addition to governing motor movements, each hemisphere appears to have a slightly different function. The dominant hemisphere (predominantly the left) is responsible for logical functions such as reasoning, number skills and scientific thought. The non-dominant right hemisphere is responsible for imagination, insight and an appreciation of shapes and their relationships, such as in 3-D forms.

For many years, people had wondered which hemisphere controlled speech. In 1836, the Frenchman Marc Dax noticed that people who suffered a paralysis of the right-hand side of their body, as a result of a stroke, frequently lost their speech as well. A paralysis of the right side of the body must be due to damage to the left hemisphere, as the left hemisphere controls the right side of the body. As the loss of speech was also due to brain damage, and as it was the left hemisphere that was damaged then, Dax deduced, it must be the left hemisphere that controls speech. Speech, then, is said to be localised in one half of the brain, usually the left hemisphere. Specifically, the production of speech is localised in Broca's area and the ability to comprehend spoken language is localised in Wernicke's area. In summary, the cerebrum is responsible for such things as reasoning ability, emotion, memory, motor movements, and speech and language skills.

Cerebellum
The cerebellum is positioned towards the back of the skull, underneath the two cerebral hemispheres. Its function is to coordinate voluntary muscle movements. If we did not have a cerebellum then any movements we made would be uncontrolled, hesitant, wavering and inaccurate. The cerebellum acts as a buffer, smoothing out any potential disruptions in our voluntary movements. It functions to help us maintain our posture and balance while we perform complex muscle movements.

Brain Stem
The brain stem is the lowest part of the brain and represents the upper extension of the spinal cord. It is concerned with automatic functions, such as heart rate, respiration, blood pressure and maintaining body temperature. It also controls reflex actions such as eye movement, and many of the drives that are necessary for survival, such as eating, sleeping and sexual activity. In addition, it acts as a sort of relay centre for sensory signals going to the cerebral cortex and motor signals coming from the cortex.

Linguistic Level (Agent)
Suppose you decide that you want to communicate to your friend that you have just seen a furry animal with four legs, whiskers on its face, a tail at its rear and sharp retractable claws. Somehow you have to encode this idea

or concept into a form that is meaningful to your friend. In English, the way you would do this is to decide upon the word *cat*. This word in English is typically used to designate the animal just described. So you have encoded a word at the linguistic level. In order to select this word it is necessary that you already have it stored in your brain. You cannot choose something that it is not available for selection. Each of us has a bank of words stored in our brains, known as our lexicon. Our lexicons are built up over time and differ from person to person. They are largely dependent upon what we have been exposed to, such as the job of work we do, where we have lived, what our interests and hobbies are, and so on. Whenever we need to encode a word we search this lexicon in order to determine whether or not we already have a word for the concept or idea we wish to convey. Selecting the appropriate word form is not necessarily an easy task.

Consider again the definition of *cat* provided above: *a furry animal with four legs, whiskers on its face, a tail at its rear and sharp retractable claws*. This definition might apply equally to *tiger, lion* or *panther*. To assist with such choices, the words in our lexicon are stored in semantic fields. These are groups of words classified by one or more similar features. For example, the word *cat* may be classified under the super-ordinate category *animal*, then in the subordinate category of *mammal* (as a sub-category of *animal*), and then the further subordinate category of *feline*. Of course, this same classification (animal-mammal-feline) could still apply equally well to a tiger, a lion or a panther. For most words in our lexicon, however, there are several levels of classification and, in the case of *cat*, it is perhaps the subordinate category of *domesticated* that distinguishes a home-loving pussy cat from the wild tigers, lions and panthers. Having selected an appropriate item from the lexicon it is usual, although not always necessary, to combine this item with other words in order to construct a meaningful utterance. There is a difference between simply uttering the word *cat* and the longer utterance *I have just seen a cat*. We have already noted that languages have specific rules that dictate which words may be combined with which other words and in what order. We have called these rules the grammar of the language. Consequently, at the linguistic level, the agent must have access to a lexicon and a set of grammatical rules.

Physiological Level (Agent)

Once the linguistic encoding has taken place, the brain sends small electrical signals along nerves from the cortex to the mouth, tongue, lips, vocal folds and the muscles which control breathing to enable us to articulate the word or words needed to communicate our thoughts. To formulate the word *cat*, you must articulate three sounds. The first is the consonant /k/, the second is the vowel /æ/ and the third is the consonant /t/ (an explanation of symbols such as these, that are used to denote speech sounds, is provided later in Chapter 6). This production of the sound sequence occurs at what is known as the physiological level and it involves rapid, coordinated, sequential movements of the vocal apparatus. The vocal apparatus consists of three parts: (1) the breathing mechanism, (2) the larynx and (3) the vocal tract.

Breathing Mechanism

In humans the chest cavity, or thorax, is separated from the abdominal cavity by a dome-shaped muscle called the diaphragm. The two lungs are enclosed within the thorax, which is supported by the ribs, and they are connected to the mouth and nose by the trachea. In an adult the trachea is about 11 cm long and 2.5 cm in diameter. It is supported by several horseshoe-shaped sections of cartilage that prevent it from collapsing and closing the airway. On inhalation the diaphragm contracts and becomes flatter as it is lowered. In addition, the lower ribs swing upwards and outwards as the external intercostal muscles contract. These movements increase the volume of the thorax and the pressure within it falls to below atmospheric pressure. Consequently, air rushes into the lungs to fill this partial vacuum. Relaxation of the external intercostals and the diaphragm allow a set of opposing muscles – the internal intercostal muscles – to return the thorax to its previous size. As the thorax diminishes in size, air is expelled from the lungs. This is known as exhalation. (Figure 1.4 shows the processes of inhalation and exhalation.) All English speech sounds are composed using exhaled air from the lungs, ie, using a pulmonic air stream.

The Larynx

The larynx is situated at the upper end of the trachea, connecting the lungs to the vocal tract. It has two main functions. The first, and most

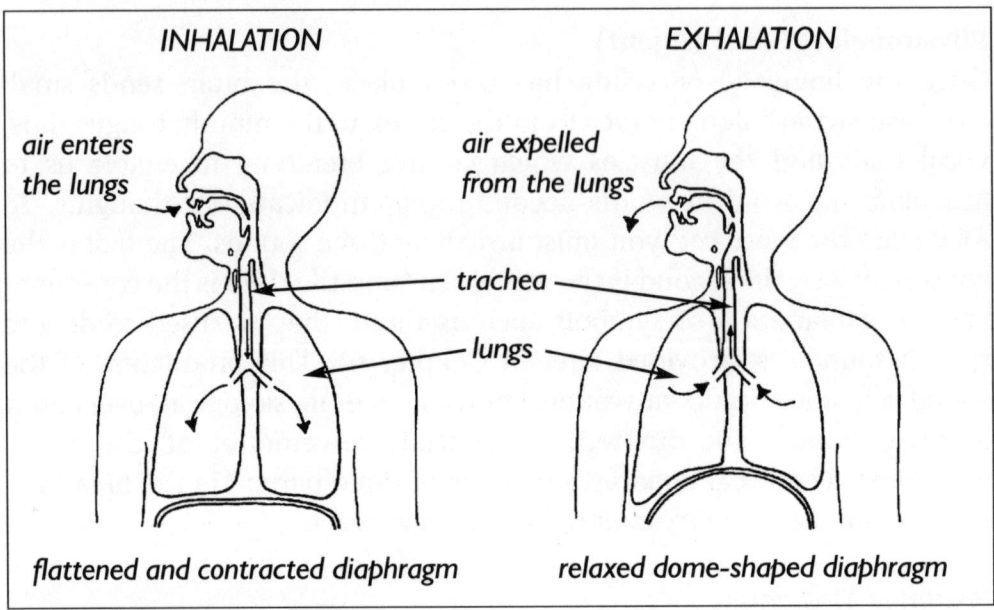

Figure 1.4 *Respiratory System*

important with respect to maintaining one's health status, is as a valve. Thus, during the act of swallowing the larynx is closed, thereby ensuring that food passes safely into the oesophagus and down into the stomach, rather than entering the lungs. The second function, and more important to the theme of this book, is as a source of sound to be used in speech.

The larynx is constructed from nine sections of cartilage. For the purpose of this discussion, however, we will restrict ourselves to a consideration of just three of these: (1) thyroid cartilage, (2) cricoid cartilage and (3) arytenoid cartilages. The thyroid cartilage is the largest of the laryngeal cartilages and forms the major chamber of the larynx. It is constructed from two relatively flat quadrilateral plates that are fused anteriorly in the midline along most of their length into a characteristic shield shape. The angle at which the plates join is different in males and females. In males it is about 90° and in females it is nearer 120°. This so-called thyroid angle is, therefore, more acute in men and is consequently more noticeable as the 'Adam's apple'. Posteriorly, each plate is extended both upwards and downwards into horns or cornu. The superior horns attach by ligaments to the hyoid bone, situated under the base of the tongue in the neck, and the inferior horns articulate with the cricoid cartilage beneath. The cricoid cartilage forms the base of the larynx. It is a complete ring of cartilage that extends upwards posteriorly to form a plate. The inferior horns of the thyroid cartilage sit on the cricoid cartilage at this posterior position. This articulation allows the cricoid cartilage to be tilted by an angle of up to 15° downwards and away from the lower anterior border of the thyroid cartilage. The cricoid cartilage is connected underneath to the upper trachea by the crico-tracheal ligament. Both the thyroid cartilage and cricoid cartilage are individual cartilages (see Figure 1.5).

The third major cartilage construction in the larynx is actually a pair of cartilages known as the arytenoid cartilages. These are pyramid-shaped and they are situated on the upper posterior part of the cricoid cartilage. One is placed laterally to the left and one laterally to the right. The arytenoids can be moved in rotational and sliding movements that are used to control the movement of the attached vocal folds. The vocal folds are approximately 17–22 mm long along their upper edge in adult males, and about 11–16 mm long in adult females. In cross-section they are almost triangular in shape. They are made of elastic tissue and are connected anteriorly to the inferior edge of the thyroid angle. Posteriorly the folds are connected to the anterior aspect of the arytenoid cartilages. Therefore, the anterior borders of the vocal folds are static, being fixed to the inner surface of the thyroid angle. As the arytenoids are variously rotated, and moved backwards and forwards, the posterior borders of the folds are either moved apart or moved close together. Air from the lungs passes upward through the trachea and through the larynx. If the vocal folds are held apart as the air passes through then the folds do not vibrate. In this position the vocal folds are said to be abducted and the space between the vocal folds is known as the glottis. When the folds are fully abducted the glottis may be up to 12 mm in width at its widest point. In contrast, the vocal folds may be held together as the air passes through, in which case they will vibrate. The vocal folds are said to be adducted when they are held together (see Figure 1.6). It is the vibration of the adducted vocal folds that creates the note on which many English speech sounds are produced. This is the human voice, and aspects of voicing in relation to speech production will be discussed in subsequent chapters. As well as lateral movements that open or close the glottis, the action of the arytenoids and the tilting of the cricoid cartilage can also increase the

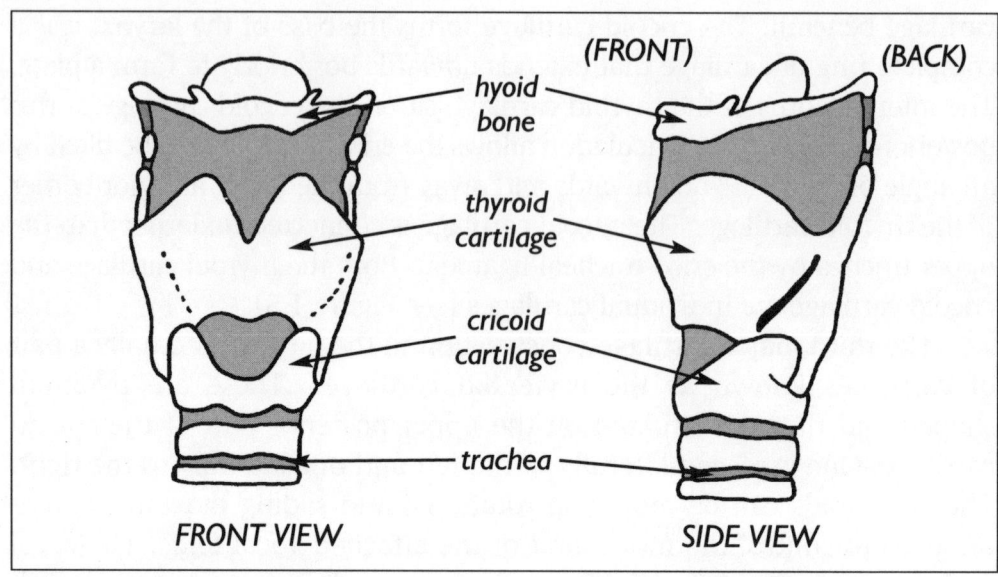

Figure 1.5 *Human Larynx*

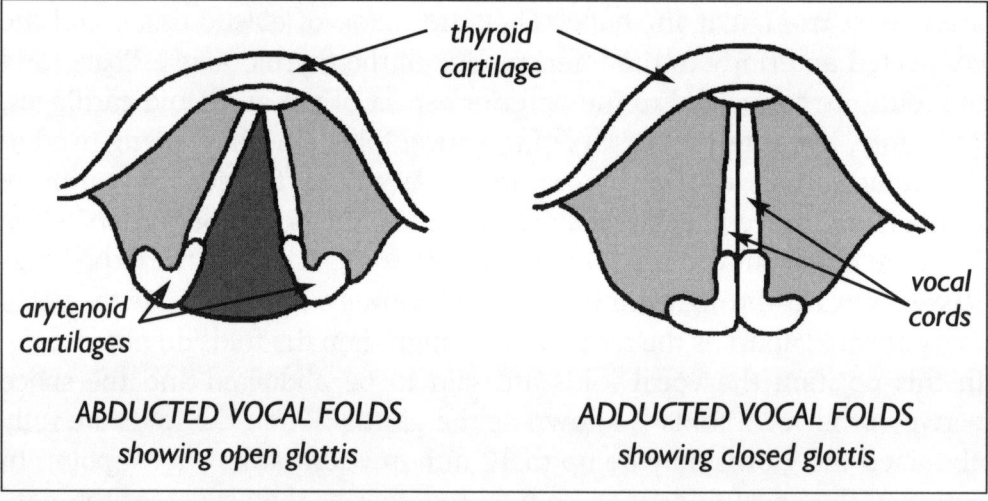

Figure 1.6 *Vocal Fold Abduction and Adduction*

tension along the length of the vocal folds. The ability to vary the tension of the folds is an important aid to varying the pitch of the voice. See Martin (1987, 7–11) and Clark & Yallop (1995, 178–186) for useful overviews of the anatomy and physiology of the larynx.

The Vocal Tract

The air passages above the larynx are known as the vocal tract. This is usually considered to be divided into two cavities: (1) the nasal cavity and (2) the oral cavity. The nasal cavity is separated from the oral cavity inferiorly by the roof of the mouth, or palate. The palate thus forms the lower surface of the nasal cavity. The upper surface is formed by soft tissue. There are no moving parts within the nasal cavity and, consequently, its overall dimensions cannot be altered. The nasal cavity extends from the nostrils to the pharynx. The pharynx is the cavity that leads from the back of the mouth and the nasal passages to the larynx and oesophagus. It is shaped somewhat like an inverted cone and may be considered as a tube of muscle that is approximately 12 cm long. Strictly, the oral cavity extends from behind the teeth to the pharynx. A third cavity, the buccal cavity, extends from behind the lips and cheeks to the front surfaces of the teeth. However, for the current purpose it is sufficient to consider the oral cavity as the area occupying the space between the lips and the pharynx.

The lower surface of the nasal cavity is the upper surface of the oral cavity, which as we have seen this consists of the palate. The front portion of the palate is a bony structure, known as the hard palate. The hard palate ends almost level with the back molars. The remaining rear portion is a flexible muscular flap, known as the soft palate, or velum. At the end of the soft palate there is a small appendage that hangs down. This is known as the uvula. It is the piece of soft, fleshy tissue that can be seen hanging down at the back of the mouth while someone continually vocalises the vowel /ɑ/ as in the words 'c<u>ar</u>', 'f<u>a</u>ther' and 'h<u>ar</u>k'. The soft palate can be raised so as to close the nasal cavity and prevent air escaping through the nose. In addition to these upper surface features, there is a bony protuberance just behind the upper incisors. This is known as the alveolar ridge. On the floor of the oral cavity is the tongue. The tongue is a large muscular organ covered by a mucous membrane that keeps it moist and lubricated. It is an extremely strong and flexible muscle. The whole upper surface of the tongue, the underside of the front portion, and the sides are all unattached and, therefore, free to move. The remainder of the tongue is attached at various places within the oral cavity. Because the oral cavity contains moving parts, the relative size and geometry of the cavity can be altered, eg, the tongue can take up different positions, the lips can be protruded or spread, the jaw can be opened or closed.

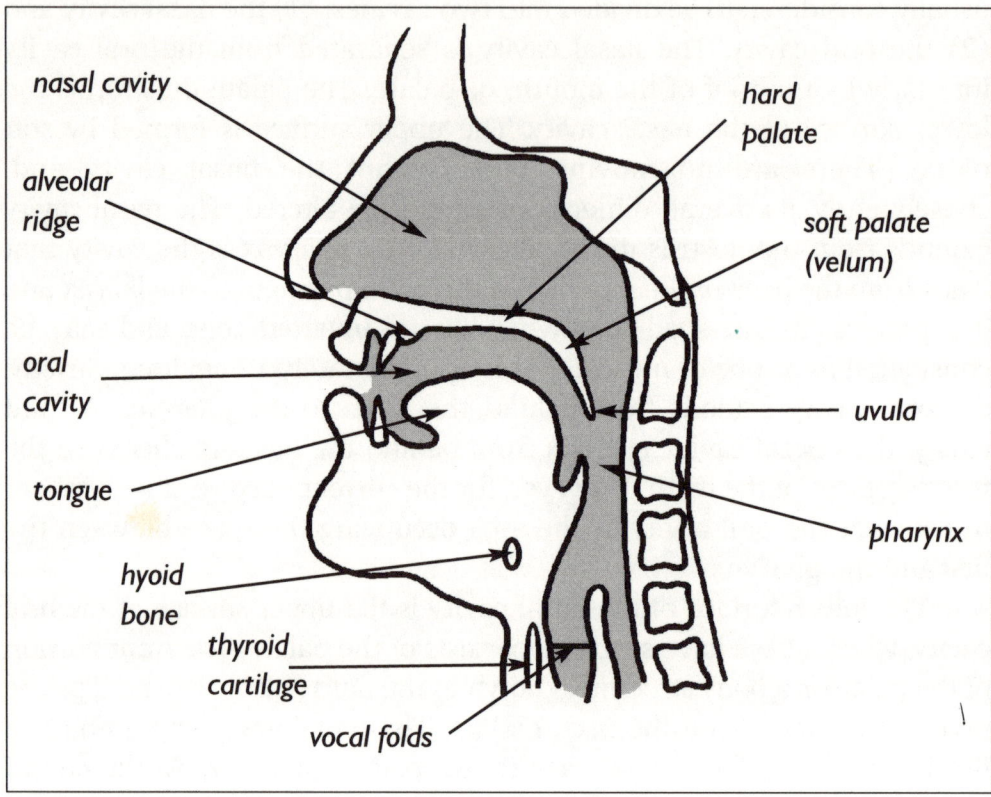

Figure 1.7 *Vocal Tract*

Feedback Loop

In order to produce clear and accurate speech, speakers must monitor their speech production. There are two ways this is achieved. The first is through sensory signals from the nerves that supply the surfaces of the tongue, lips, palate and other parts of the vocal apparatus. The transmission of signals through the nervous system allows the speaker to monitor, for example, where the various parts of the vocal apparatus are in 3-D space in relation to each other. This is known as proprioceptive feedback. The second – and perhaps more important means – is through auditory feedback. As we speak we are continually listening for any errors in our production and making the necessary modifications.

Acoustic Level

The movements of the vocal apparatus produce changes in the surrounding air. The atoms that compose the air are disturbed and each atom bumps into an adjacent one, which in turn bumps into the next one, and so on. This rhythmic disturbance of air is known as a speech sound wave; it travels through the air from the speaker's mouth to the ear of the listener. The speech sound wave occurs at what is known as the acoustic level.

Physiological Level (Recipient)

When the speech sound wave arrives at the listener's ear it causes their eardrum, or tympanic membrane, to vibrate. This, in turn, causes the movement of three small bones (ossicles) within the middle ear: the malleus or hammer, the incus or anvil, and the stapes or stirrup (see Figure 1.8). Their function is to amplify the vibration of the sound wave.

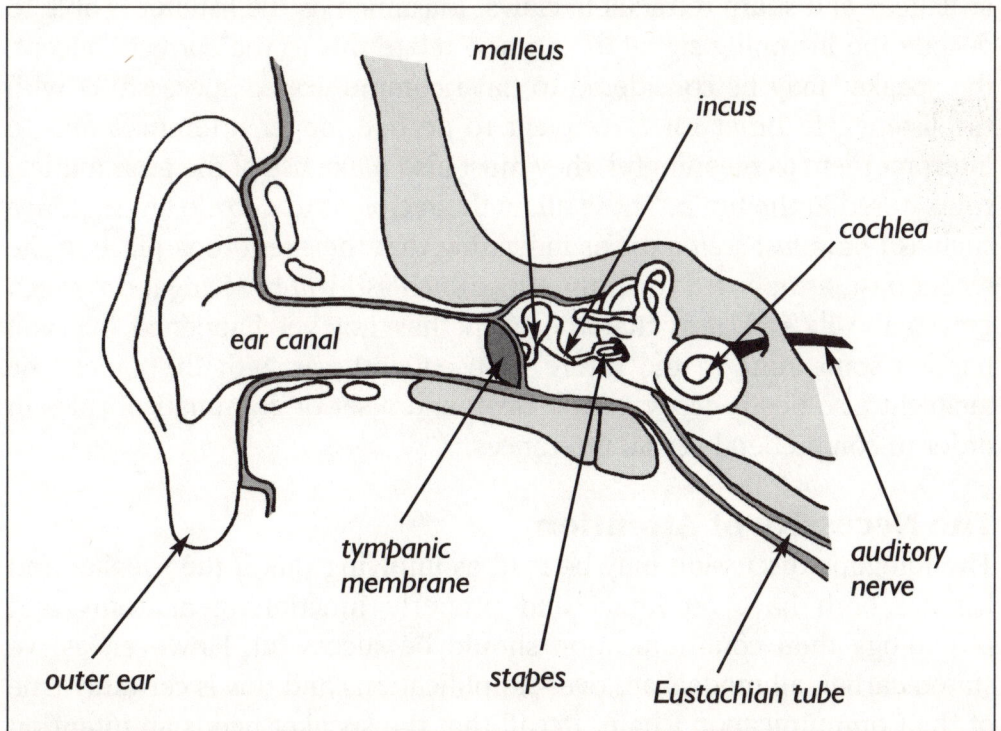

Figure 1.8 *The Ear*

The stapes is, in turn, connected to a membrane in the wall of the cochlea. The cochlea is designed to convert the vibrations into electrical signals that are subsequently transmitted along the auditory nerve to the brain of the listener. Again, this takes place at what is known as the physiological level. (For a succinct overview of the anatomy and physiology of the head and neck and the respiratory system see Martini & Welch, 1999.)

Linguistic Level (Recipient)
The listener then unravels and decodes the electrical impulses from the cochlea in the cortex and reforms them into the word or words of the message, again at the linguistic level. If the incoming signals are decoded into the single word *cat*, for example, the listener compares this with other words in their own lexicon. The listener is then able to determine that the word is a proper word and that it represents, in this example, the concept of a furry (domesticated) animal with four legs, whiskers on its face, a tail at its rear and sharp retractable claws. Inasmuch as the listener is able to decode the incoming signal as *cat*, and relate this to the correct concept, the speaker may be considered to have communicated successfully with the listener. In order for a recipient to decode longer utterances and to interpret them as meaningful, they must also make use of the grammatical rules stored in the brain. These allow the recipient to decode an utterance such as *I have just seen a cat* as indicating that the event took place in the recent past, as opposed to an utterance such as *I will be seeing a cat* which grammatically indicates that the event has not yet happened but will happen some time in the future. Consequently, as with the agent, the recipient also needs access to a lexicon and a set of grammatical rules in order to comprehend verbal utterances.

The Necessity of Attention
The foregone discussion may be read as implying that if the speaker and listener both have an intact and properly functioning anatomy and physiology then communication should be successful. However, as we stated earlier, all models are over-simplifications and this is certainly true of the Communication Chain. Recall that the speaker needs an intention to communicate. Similarly, the recipient needs an intention to receive the

speaker's utterances. What do we mean by this? Well, consider a recipient who has an intact hearing system. In other words, when sound waves hit the recipient's eardrum the vibrations of the eardrum are appropriately converted into electrical signals which are subsequently transmitted to the recipient's brain. However, this does not necessarily mean that the recipient will interpret or understand the utterance. This is because there is a difference between hearing an utterance and listening to an utterance. I may be physiologically capable of hearing the speech sound wave, but unless I actively attend to it, and attempt to understand, then I am not listening. You will, no doubt, be familiar with the situation where you have been talking at length to someone and then have broken up your flow of conversation to ask, 'Are you listening to me?' You know that the recipient is capable of hearing you, but you are suspicious that they are not actually listening. We are surrounded with sound all the time, of course. Stop for a moment right now, put down this reading material and listen to the sounds in your present environment. What can you hear? Is there a bird singing? A door or a floorboard creaking? A child giggling? The sound of your own breathing? Music in the background? Leaves rustling outside your window? Traffic noises in the distance? The chances are that until you stopped and actively attended to these sounds you were unaware of them – despite the fact that they may have been going on for some time. We are in this state for much of the time, of course. Most of us, however, have learnt to filter out sounds that are currently unimportant. It is only when we attend to a sound that we become aware of it. Thus, for communication to be successful, as well as the speaker demonstrating an intention to transmit an utterance, the recipient must also attend to that utterance, ie, listen to it. Taking account of the necessity for attention, we should now amend our summary definition of communication to read:

Human communication is an intentional act performed by a human agent for the purpose of causing some effect in an attentive human recipient.

Conversation

The above definition, while accurate, does not fully emphasise the two-way nature of human communication. Indeed, the model of communication as presented in the Communication Chain encourages us to focus on a single act of communication from one agent to one recipient. However, communication is a reciprocal social activity. In most everyday, informal interactions it would be unusual for just one participant to take the full burden of transmitting information to another without some feedback on that information, or without also receiving some information in return. In reality the roles of agent and recipient are constantly alternating. At one moment I may be the agent who is instigating a verbal utterance. Upon completion of the utterance, however, I may then become the recipient, as the former recipient takes on the role of agent and responds verbally to my immediately prior utterance. There is a constant interplay between the participants, with each taking turns at either instigating a verbal utterance or acting as an attentive recipient. This reciprocal, interactive discourse is known as conversation. Indeed, conversation is the archetypal language use by which people participate in social interactions. In Chapter 9 we will consider some of the characteristics of conversation and examine how conversational participants manage conversations in real time. For now, this concludes our overview of the nature of human communication. In the next chapter we commence our exploration of language.

Revision Exercises

1.1 What is the difference between language, speech and non-verbal communication?

1.2 List three prerequisite skills for the development of language, and three for the development of speech.

1.3 What are the three major links in the Communication Chain?

1.4 With respect to the Communication Chain, describe the different processes that take place at the linguistic level of the agent and that of the recipient.

Activities

1.5 Observe an adult in conversation with another person. Identify and list the various non-verbal communication components that are used. Do these components serve to enhance or lessen the effectiveness of communication? How?

1.6 Find a busy public place where you can sit relatively unobtrusively, but where you can eavesdrop on the talk that is taking place (such as in a café). Make a list of the reasons why the people there are communicating. Do the people have only one purpose that continues throughout the whole conversation? How frequently does the purpose change? Do the people engaged in conversation explicitly declare their purpose, or have you had to infer the purpose from what was said?

1.7 Observe a conversation between two people for at least 10 minutes. Keep a count of how many utterances (turns at talking) are made by each participant. How often do the roles of agent and recipient alternate? Does one participant take more of an agent's role? Is one participant more passive, taking a predominantly recipient role? Explain your findings.

Note

1 *Throughout this book, when it is necessary to specify a precise age, we will adopt the convention of citing ages in years and months, separated by a semi-colon. For example, for a person aged five years and five months, this will be written as 5;05 years. For a person aged seven years and eleven months, this will be formulated as 7;11 years.*

CHAPTER 2

Language Properties, Acquisition & Development

THIS CHAPTER INTRODUCES PART 2 of the book and begins our examination of language. We consider three issues: the key properties of language, its acquisition, and its development. We start with a consideration of how to define language and then highlight eight key properties: arbitrariness, duality, systematicity, structure-dependence, productivity, displacement, specialisation, and cultural transmission. Then we make a distinction between general language ability and the ability to use a particular world language. Next, we consider possible answers to the question, how do humans acquire language skills? Specifically, four possibilities are outlined: probability, imitation, cognition and innate ability. The debate as to whether or not animals have, or are capable of using, language is touched on briefly during our discussion of innate ability. We conclude the chapter with a description of the development of early language from pre-linguistic vocalisations, through the Early One Word Stage and on to the Complex Utterance Stage, typically achieved at around 5;00 years of age.

What is Language?
Linguistics is the scientific study of language and you might suppose that, because it *is* scientific, then there would be no difficulty in defining

language. You do not have to have read much about science to realise that scientists differ in their definitions and interpretations of the 'facts'. There are, of course, some general observations to which all investigators subscribe, for example:

Language is the predominant means by which human beings communicate with each other.
Language is the means by which humans organise their societies.

However, such high-level observations are insufficient to describe the intricacies and peculiarities of language. The difficulty is that because researchers are interested in different facets of a subject, and because of the complexity of language itself, there is no one universally accepted definition. Most attempts to define language, therefore, result in the construction of lists of characteristics of language (Hockett, 1963; Linden, 1974). The problem with this approach, however, is in determining how many characteristics are minimally sufficient to describe language. Two characteristics? Four? Twenty? In addition, as Aitchison (1976, 36) points out: 'to use [a] list to define language is like trying to define a man by noting that he has two arms, two legs, a head, a belly button, he bleeds if you scratch him, and shrieks if you tread on his toe'. However, having accepted the shortfalls of this procedure, an outline of essential characteristics does appear to be the best way forward at present. As indicated, there are many so-called key properties of language, but we will confine ourselves to an outline of just eight: (1) arbitrariness, (2) duality, (3) systematicity, (4) structure-dependence, (5) productivity, (6) displacement, (7) specialisation, and (8) cultural transmission.

Arbitrariness
Essentially, language is a symbol system. In broad terms, the symbols of language are words. By constructing words and stringing them together according to a set of rules – the grammar of the language – we are able to construct meaningful utterances. The choice of symbols used by a language is, however, said to be arbitrary. This is because there is no direct relationship between a particular word and its meaning. For example, in English we use the word *cup* to represent a physical object

capable of holding liquids, which usually has a handle, and which humans use to drink from. Of course, there is no particular reason why we should use the word-symbol *cup*. We could just as easily choose to use the word *zarg*, or *pinkt*, or any other word form we might think of. The point is that words are just an arbitrary set of symbols used to represent various meanings. In summary, if we know the form of a word it is impossible to predict the meaning, and if we know the meaning it is impossible to predict the form. Each particular language (English, French, Russian, Chinese, etc) uses a different set of symbols. So, for example, the word-symbol for *cup* in French is *tasse*, but in Portuguese it is *chávena*. Arbitrariness is a useful property because it increases the flexibility of language. The flexibility arises because language is not constrained by the need to match the form of a word and its meaning. Therefore it is possible to construct an almost infinite number of words from a limited set of speech sounds. Having made the point that linguistic symbols are arbitrary, there are some English words that appear to be less arbitrary than others. These are onomatopoeic words – that is, words that imitate the sound associated with an object or an action. For example, in the utterance *the bees were buzzing* the word *buzzing* actually sounds like the noise bees make. Other examples include *hiss* and *rasp*. The features of such words are often exploited in the writing of poetry.

Duality

Language appears to be organised at least at two levels. The primary level consists of the units and the secondary level consists of the elements. The elements of the secondary level combine to form the units of the primary level. For our purposes, we can consider the elements of verbal language to be speech sounds, ie, consonants and vowels. These speech sounds then combine to form units at the primary level, ie, words. We saw in the first chapter how the word *cat* is formed by the combination of three speech sounds: the consonant /k/, the vowel /æ/ and the consonant /t/. These speech sounds at the primary level are meaningless if they are uttered in isolation. For example, if I just say the sound /k/ this has no meaning. Similarly, /æ/ and /t/ spoken on their own are meaningless. It is only when these secondary-level elements are combined in a systematic way that they have the possibility of conveying meaning. Consequently, *cat* /kæt/ is meaningful, whereas /k/ and /æ/ and /t/ are not.

Systematicity

Language is an orderly method of communicating ideas, thoughts, emotions, and so on. If language were random then there would be no way of ensuring that the intended meaning was conveyed. Regularity and order are essential for language to work properly. We have seen an example of this above when considering duality. We noted that the secondary level elements /k/, /æ/ and /t/ may combine to form the primary level unit *cat* /kæt/. These three elements may also be recombined to form the word *act* /ækt/. However, the combination /æ/ + /t/ + /k/ to form *atc* /ætk/ is meaningless. What this demonstrates is that language is governed by rules that define which combinations of elements are acceptable and which are not. There are also rules that govern the combination of primary level units. So, for example, we realise that the utterance *the first snows of winter* is appropriate, whereas the combination *snows winter first the of* is not.

Structure-Dependence

Language appears to have an underlying patterned structure, and humans appear to be able to recognise these patterns intuitively. Consider the following utterance:

the very happy man from Billingham	kissed	the shy woman

We intuitively realise that this utterance patterns into coherent segments. This is demonstrated by the fact that we are able to easily remove one segment and replace it with another, for example:

he	kissed	the shy woman
the very happy man from Billingham	kissed	her
Graham	kissed	Margaret

As well as recognising that we can substitute one segment with another, further evidence that we intuitively recognise patterns in language is demonstrated by our ability to restructure segments readily. Consider again our opening utterance:

the very happy man from Billingham	kissed	the shy woman

This utterance could be restructured as follows:

the shy woman	was kissed by	the very happy man from Billingham

We are able to recognise that this latter utterance is the structural equivalent of the former utterance. Of course, the patterned structure of language allows us to both rearrange and substitute segments simultaneously, for example:

she	was kissed by	the very happy man from Billingham
the shy woman	was kissed by	him
Margaret	was kissed by	Graham

Productivity

Many animals respond to stimuli in their environment in predictable ways. For example, the stimulus of seeing a collection of shiny objects in front of a small grass covert will stimulate a female Bowerbird to mate with the male bird who prepared the display. The sight of the objects stimulates the female to perform a particular behaviour, in this case pairing and mating. Similarly, the stimulus of cold weather and reduced daylight hours stimulates the ground squirrel to perform a certain behaviour – hibernation. These behaviours, and others like them, are said to be stimulus-bound. In other words, if we know what the stimulus is then we can predict the subsequent behaviour. The behaviour is invariant and always follows a specific stimulus.

If language were stimulus-bound we would expect that each time a human was presented with the same stimulus they would utter exactly the same words. Clearly this is not so. If three people were all shown the painting *Mona Lisa* there is no guarantee that each would utter the same words. A variety of responses are available to these people. They may be just as likely to say something along the lines of 'What a beautiful picture', as they are 'That reminds me of my sister', or 'Oh, I've forgotten to put the kettle on!' The salient point is that it is not possible to predict that a particular stimulus will cause a human to use one, and only one, particular language construction. In this sense, language is said to be stimulus-free, and this explains why humans are able to use language creatively. Language is, therefore, flexible.

The fact that language is stimulus-free and flexible leads to the notion of productivity – ie, that language can be used to construct an infinite set of new and meaningful utterances. These utterances are novel in that they may never have been spoken before and yet they are meaningful and readily interpretable by other people.

Displacement

Language also allows us to think of, and communicate about, something or someone that is not immediately present. So, for example, we can refer to our new car even though it is not actually in front of us. Similarly, we can discuss last night's football game even though it has passed. This property of language is known as displacement.

Specialisation

This key property refers to the fact that language allows us to substitute an arbitrary word for a physical action. An example might be a child who instructs a friend to 'Stay away!'. This utterance means that the child does not then have to act out the message, for example, by physically pushing the friend away. Similarly, the police officer who instructs a crowd to 'Move along!' has used language to substitute for the physical action of driving the crowd forwards. In both instances language has substituted for a physical action.

Cultural Transmission

Language is the means by which humans are able to teach the younger generation all that they have learned to date. It is the primary, and most efficient, method of transmitting necessary knowledge, experiences and social norms of behaviour to each successive generation. One of the most obvious examples of this is the formal teaching in our schools, the majority of which is undertaken using verbal language. The child who sits on its parent's knee and listens to stories of family traditions and events is also learning through language. This property of language is referred to as cultural transmission. The language of a particular society, therefore, forms part of the culture of that society.

Langage et Langue

Following on from the above discussion it is necessary to make a further point. It is important to distinguish between language in general and a particular language. The distinction is not so obvious in English because we only use the one word *language* to describe both aspects. In French, however, the word *langage* is used to mean language in general – ie, the possession of a language capacity and, by inference, the knowledge that allows us to learn any particular language. It is this possession of language ability that is most often thought of as the distinguishing feature between animals and humans. By comparison, the French word *langue* is used to refer to a particular language – eg, English, Indonesian, Hindi, Swedish. Therefore, it should be apparent that in order to learn and speak a particular language – English, Indonesian or whatever – you need to possess language – ie, have the necessary linguistic skills to manipulate the symbols of the particular language. It is a matter of fate that we learn a particular language. We just happen to have been born in the UK, or Indonesia, or somewhere else. Therefore we learn the particular language(s) spoken in the place where we grow up (*langue*). However, we all have the capacity to learn any particular language because we possess general language-learning skills (*langage*). In other words, there is nothing special about the brains of English-speaking people that makes them different from, say, people who speak Indonesian. If the English child and Indonesian child had been swapped at birth, such that each grew up in the other's home country, then they would have learnt the language(s) indigenous to that country. This is because they both possess language in general (*langage*).

Language Acquisition

One of the most interesting questions is, how do humans acquire language skills? As with attempts to define language, there is again no universally accepted explanation. Several answers have been proposed, however, and we will consider four of them in the following subsections: (1) probability, (2) imitation, (3) cognition, and (4) innate ability.

Probability

A possible explanation for the way children learn language is based on a mathematical model of probability or chance. Consider the fact that certain words nearly always occur together. For example, *bread* and *butter*, *fish* and *chips*. Because these words frequently occur together, in preference to other words such as *bread* and *plaster* or *fish* and *typewriter*, they are said to collocate highly. Words do associate with more than one other word, however. For example, the word *chips* also occurs in association with *microcomputers* (if we are referring to silicone chips). As these two words do not occur together as frequently as *fish* and *chips* they are still said to collocate, but less highly. Thus, the probability theory of language learning asserts that as children are exposed to language they learn to associate those words that occur together most frequently, and therefore are able to construct the rules of speaking and generate sequences of meaningful utterances. One main criticism of this theory is that it offers no explanation as to how children use language creatively – ie, how they can say totally new and novel things. If a child is shown a photograph of its mother, the child is just as likely to say, 'That's my mum!', as 'Nice picture!', or any number of other things. Relying on the statistical probability of one word associating itself strongly with another does not add much to our understanding of these sorts of situations. This aspect of language was referred to earlier when, during our discussion of the key property of productivity, we noted that language is stimulus-free.

Imitation

Historically, the most famous proponent of the so-called imitation theory of language learning is the Harvard psychologist BF Skinner (1957). In brief, this theory proposes that the child hears what the adults in its environment are saying and simply copies what is heard. The child also learns to associate certain things it has heard with particular events. So the child may hear, 'It's a drink', while at the same time being handed a beaker of orange juice. In this way it is thought that the child learns the meaning of the words it hears. Similarly, if the child makes an attempt to communicate, for example by saying 'di' and, at the same time pointing to a cup, the parent is likely to reward this attempt by giving the child a drink. Thus, the child learns through imitation, association and reinforcement. This process is sometimes known as learning theory. The one overriding difficulty with this theory is that everyday language does not provide a very good model of 'correct' adult speech. Adults are always tripping over their words, hesitating, using slang and regional dialects. If you want proof of this, listen very carefully to the structure of what is being said and write down some examples next time you are in the company of a few adults. How, then, could the child possibly sift through this mass of confused signals to imitate only those words and phrases that reflect 'correct' speech? In addition, an examination of the types of mistakes children make demonstrates that they are attempting to apply rules to their language, and not simply to copy adults (Ervin-Tripp, 1964). Consider the following child's utterance:

mummy goed home

The first thing to notice is that this cannot be an imitation of an adult's utterance, as adults do not speak in this manner. The second point is that the child appears to be attempting to apply some sort of linguistic rule. Instead of using the correct past tense form *went*, the child appears to be attempting to make the verb *go* into a past tense by the addition of the suffix *-ed*. This is the appropriate strategy for verbs such as *walk* and *pray*, which become *walked* and *prayed* respectively. However, the child appears to have over-generalised this rule on this occasion. The important point, though, is that the child produces an utterance that clearly cannot be an imitation of an adult model, and which also shows evidence of being governed by some rule system.

Cognition

A cognitive theory tries to get 'inside' the mind of the child and to propose the types of mental structures and thinking processes that may be taking place. It is argued that the child cannot move on to learning a new language skill until it is intellectually ready for the next stage. This theory was most forcefully presented by the Swiss psychologist Jean Piaget (1952). He argued that children have to have a certain psychological capacity, or cognitive ability, before they can learn particular aspects of using language in order to make themselves understood. One example of this is that children must have the mental ability to appreciate that people or things still exist even when they are out of sight. If they cannot appreciate this, then it would be very difficult, for example, for the child to understand and respond appropriately to questions such as, 'Where is your dad?', when the child is at nursery school and the father is at work. The child must have the mental ability to understand that dad still exists, and that he exists in some place away from the nursery, in order to explain where he is. This cognitive ability is known as object permanence. At face value, cognitive theory appears to be intuitively correct. After all, a 16;00-year-old is able to learn and play the game of chess more readily than a 5;00-year-old. As the game of chess requires good analytic and predictive capacities, the more intellectually able 16;00-year-old is better suited to learning its intricacies. By extension, if the acquisition of language is solely dependent upon intellectual ability then, according to cognitive theory, one might reasonably predict that older children would learn a new language more easily than younger children, as they are intellectually more able. While learning the rules of chess is simpler for the 16;00-year-old child's superior intellect, research has shown that the 5;00-year-old child would learn a foreign language more easily than the older adolescent (see Brown, 1958; Lenneberg, 1967; Curtis *et al*, 1974). Consequently, the acquisition of language cannot be quite as straightforward as being solely related to a developing intellect – if it were, then the 16;00-year-old should learn the new language more easily.

Innate Ability

The innatist theory states that human beings are genetically pre-programmed to learn language, that they have an innate ability to learn the languages that exist in the world. While many researchers have promoted this view, it has been popularised most effectively by the American linguist Noam Chomsky (1965; 1972). The assertion that humans are predisposed to learn language is argued on several counts. We will discuss four of these here: (1) the structure of human speech organs, (2) language is unique to humans, (3) the speed of acquisition of language, and (4) the existence of linguistic universals.

The Structure of Human Speech Organs

In describing the anatomy of the human brain, respiratory system and vocal tract in the preceding chapter, we did not contrast this with the anatomy of other animals. Had we done so the differences would have become especially apparent, and the uniqueness of the human vocal apparatus unequivocal. Humans are most often compared with apes and, in fact, our vocal apparatus is extraordinarily similar to that found in all mammals. The uniqueness, however, has more to do with the location of the organs and, especially, the larynx. In humans the larynx is located lower down in the neck. The consequence of this is that it increases the area available for us to modify sounds. The ability to produce certain sounds is unique to humans. For example, only humans can produce the consonant sounds /k/ as in *kite* and /g/ as in *gun*, and the vowel sounds /ɒ/ as in *hot*, /i/ as in *beet*, and /u/ as in *shoe*. Moreover, apes do not have the necessary fine control over the diaphragm and other muscles involved in breathing which allows humans voluntarily to use air from the lungs for speech.

We have recognised that to communicate orally we need both an appropriate vocal apparatus and a brain capable of processing large amounts of symbolic information. In humans we can identify a language centre in both hemispheres of the brain, within what is known as the planum temporale. In 94 per cent of people, the part of the brain known as Wernicke's area, situated within the planum temporale, is larger in the left hemisphere than in the right. For these people, the left hemisphere is the dominant side for language. Until very recently it was thought that no language centre was located in the brains of the great apes. However, in

1998 a research team from the Mount Sinai School of Medicine led by Patrick Gannon (Gannon *et al*, 1998) made surface measurements of the size of the planum temporale in 18 chimpanzee brains. Their findings showed that in 17 out of the 18 chimp brains the area was larger in the left hemisphere than in the right, ie, 94 per cent – just as in humans. This finding is obviously not conclusive, but it does suggest the possibility that humans and chimps may share a common neurological substrate for language. In addition to this language-processing part of the brain, we also know that humans are adept at processing auditory signals. At about one month of age a human infant is capable of distinguishing between certain speech sounds, such as /p/ as in the word *pin*; /b/ as in the word *bin*; /t/ as in the word *tin*, and /d/ as in the word *din*. At just six months of age the infant is capable of detecting sounds as quiet as one decibel (dB) (for comparison, a whisper is around 10 dB). Human infants also appear to be capable of detecting differences between speech sounds used in their own native language (eg, English, French, Vietnamese) and those used in other languages. This suggests that humans' auditory perception is genetically pre-programmed and indicates an innate preparedness to learn language.

Language is Unique to Humans
While no one would disagree that the human compulsion to communicate is realised by their use of language, some have challenged the claim that language can be used only by humans. One of the most famous people to query this view was Samuel Pepys. Writing about a 'baboone' in his diary in 1661 he commented, 'I do believe it already understands much English; and I am of the mind it might be taught to speak or make signs' (cited in Wallman, 1992, 11). In more recent times, attempts have been made to teach language skills to a variety of animals, but most success has been achieved through working with chimpanzees. The two most famous chimps were Washoe (Gardner & Gardner, 1969) and Sarah (Premack, 1970; 1971), who began their training in the 1960s.

We have already noted that while a chimpanzee's anatomy is similar to that of a human, it does not have the requisite vocal apparatus to be able to speak. Because of this, Washoe was taught a version of American Sign Language and Sarah was taught to manipulate plastic tokens on a magnetic board. While both were able to learn some aspects of language, the process was extremely slow and laborious and, in the case of Washoe, resulted in a vocabulary of only 85 signs and 294 two-sign combinations after about five years' training. It is quite an understatement to say that this does not compare with the extensive development in language skills achieved by the average 5;00-year-old human. However, both Washoe and Sarah demonstrated some of the key properties of language. With respect to Washoe, a remarkable development occurred when she adopted an infant chimp named Loulis. No sign language was used by humans in Loulis' presence for five years, and yet Loulis was able to learn over 50 signs through her association with Washoe. This demonstrates the property of cultural transmission, ie, the chimps continued to use sign language and pass this on to other chimps without any input from humans (Gardner & Gardner, 1989).

Sarah was also able to demonstrate displacement. She was presented with the construction 'Brown (is the) colour of chocolate' when there was no chocolate in sight. Later, she was shown several coloured objects and presented with the phrase, 'Take brown', and she successfully selected a brown object (Premack, 1976). Therefore Sarah was able to use language to think of something that was not immediately present and to apply that learning at a later time.

Several other apes have been taught language skills, and in the 1970s it was reported that a chimp named Nim was able to demonstrate the key language property of specialisation – ie, rather than acting out messages, the speaker is able to use an arbitrary word. Nim, who was also taught to sign, would sign the warning *bite* and *angry* to express discontent if he was preparing to attack. He would, however, not attack if he perceived that his warning was heeded. This demonstrates how Nim was able to substitute an arbitrary 'word' (*bite-angry*) for a physical action (Terrace, 1979). Further, in 1994 it was reported that an ape known as Kanzi was able to demonstrate the key property of productivity. Kanzi was alleged to have learnt certain signs by observing its mother and eventually learnt to create new signs, such as *drink-fruit* for 'watermelon' (Savage-Rumbaugh & Lewin, 1994). We see, then, that these chimps were able to demonstrate some of the key properties of language. It is worth noting, however, that even if an animal could be taught to use language this does not imply that it is genetically pre-programmed to acquire language. For comparison, it may be possible to teach a human how to dig a rabbit's burrow, but this does not prove that humans are genetically pre-programmed to do so. In summary, chimpanzees are able to learn some of the rudiments of language, but they do not appear to be predisposed to this.

The Speed of Acquisition of Language
Innatists argue that the staggering rate at which children acquire language skills can only be explained if one supposes that children are genetically pre-programmed to learn language. They contest that the child does not come to the language-learning task with a blank mind – *tabula rasa* – but has an innate disposition to learn language. This claim is put into perspective when we note that the average 5;00-year-old has an expressive vocabulary of around 2,000 words, and that by the age of 7;00 years this will have doubled. In addition, the size of the comprehension vocabulary (ie, the words understood by the child, but not necessarily used expressively) will be much higher than this. Further, a 5;00-year-old will be using near-adult sentence constructions and all but the most difficult speech sounds. Moreover, the child will be able to use language for a variety of reasons: to express feelings, to make requests, to disagree and so on. This is a remarkable feat to which chimps may never aspire.

Linguistic Universals and Language
Innatists noted that while different languages (eg, English, Welsh, Chinese, Russian) all have different rules or grammars, they also have many things in common. These language similarities are known as linguistic universals. We will consider just two examples here: negatives and relative clauses.

A well-documented example of a linguistic universal is the way children develop the use of negatives (Klima & Bellugi, 1966). With respect to this, it has been shown that children follow remarkably similar routes when learning a language. They seem to follow a predetermined pattern of language-learning through which all normally developing children pass. At around 1;06 years children learning English form utterances made up of two-word combinations such as the following:

daddy gone
Sarah play
doggy bark

At first, when they attempt to make the utterances negative, children simply put *no* or *not* in front of the two-word combination:

no daddy gone
not Sarah play
no doggy bark

At a later stage the child appears to realise that the negative should be contained within the utterance, and the *no* or *not* is then inserted between the words:

daddy *no* gone
Sarah *not* play
doggy *no* bark

Eventually the true adult form is used:

daddy *did not* go
Sarah *is not* playing
the dog *is not* barking

The important point to note here is that, with the obvious exception of the true adult forms, the child could not possibly have been imitating adult utterances. This is because the child's utterances do not represent grammatical English constructions. In short, adults do not talk like this!

The linguists Neil Smith and Deirdre Wilson (1979) cite what are known as 'relative clauses' as a further example of a linguistic universal. They do this on the basis that, among the many world languages, there are only two principal procedures for constructing such clauses. Briefly, a relative clause is a phrase within an utterance that refers back to the head noun of the utterance. For example, in the construction *the play that I like* the relative clause is *that I like*, as the *that* refers back to the head noun of the utterance, *play*. It is not really important to understand this concept fully at this stage, as the relative clauses are shown in capital letters in the following examples. The first strategy for forming relative clauses is exemplified by languages such as English:

the film THAT YOU SAW
the man THAT YOU CALLED
the woman THAT YOU LOVE

The second important method is exemplified by languages such as Hebrew. These languages insert an additional pronoun (eg, *it*, *him*, *her*) into the clause:

the film THAT YOU SAW IT
the man THAT YOU CALLED HIM
the woman THAT YOU LOVE HER

In theory, it would be possible to construct relative clauses in any number of different ways. However, the fact that most languages in the world adopt one of these two methods is in itself quite remarkable. It is a good example of a linguistic universal.

Language acquisition device (LAD)
Chomsky (1972) refers to the child's innate general language-learning ability as the Language Acquisition Device (LAD). He claims that children have a blueprint in the brain that allows them to recognise the structure-dependence of language, and to manipulate these structures. Consider the following utterance:

Graham kissed Margaret

We have already noted in our earlier consideration of the structure-dependence of language that the larger units of language can be both substituted and manipulated to produce utterances such as the following:

Margaret was kissed by Graham

When we consider these two utterances it is apparent that they both have the same meaning. However, their form, or structure, is different. We would say, therefore, that they both have the same deep structure, but that they have a different surface structure. The original utterance *Graham kissed Margaret* could also be manipulated to form the following utterances:

Who Graham kissed was Margaret
The person kissed by Graham was Margaret
It was Margaret who Graham kissed

Again, we must conclude that each of these utterances has the same meaning, or deep structure (ie, *Graham kissed Margaret*), but that their surface structures are quite different. Now consider the following utterance:

the chicken was ready to eat

What is the deep structure of this utterance? This is much harder to determine because the utterance is ambiguous. The possible deep structures may be represented diagrammatically as follows:

the chicken was ready	for	the chicken to eat for itself

the chicken was ready	for	someone to eat the chicken

On the basis of the utterance alone, we are uncertain as to whether or not the chicken is ready to eat for itself or if the chicken is ready to be eaten by someone else. In this instance, therefore, we see that two different deep structures give rise to just the one surface structure. Now consider the following utterances:

the chicken was anxious to eat
the chicken was delicious to eat

The syntax of these two utterances is alike. Structurally, therefore, they are akin and they are again said to have a similar surface structure. However, their meanings are quite different. In the case of the first utterance it is the chicken that is doing the eating. In the second utterance it is the chicken that is being eaten! Consequently, while these two utterances demonstrate a similar, but not exactly the same, surface structure they have different deep structures. Chomsky argues that children 'know' about deep structures and that they are able to apply rules that allow them to manipulate these structures, giving rise to a variety of surface structures. He calls these grammatical rules *transformations*.

Chomsky's ideas in relation to language acquisition are persuasive and his theories have gained ground over the years. In sum, his proposals seem to imply that if a child has a properly functioning LAD then language will develop regardless of the kinds of experience the child is exposed to. Alternatively, if the LAD is damaged in some way it would seem that no amount of environmental support or teaching would make a difference. However, two main criticisms may be made. First, rather like the cognitive theories, the innatist view tends to focus on the 'inside' mental structures and thinking processes of the child. It is unlikely, therefore, that what research evidence we might be able to gather would enable us to understand fully exactly what is going on inside a child's mind. However, researchers have developed techniques for making informed inferences from what they observe. Second, and perhaps more important, the role of other people in assisting the child to learn language tends to be overlooked. As noted in the discussion of the imitation theory of language acquisition, adult speech is fraught with hesitations, repetitions, slips of the tongue, etc, and it therefore provides an imperfect model. However, research has shown that adults do in fact make considerable modifications to their speech when talking to children (Ringler, 1981). These modifications are designed to assist the child with language-learning and this type of modified talk is often referred to as 'motherese'.

Motherese
It has long been known that mothers demonstrate a style of speaking to their babies that is uncommonly different from their normal adult conversation. This is also true of those who have worked with young infants for some time. Researchers have investigated this so-called motherese and discovered that all cultures have some form of baby talk (Slobin, 1967; Drach, 1969). Up to a child's first birthday the mother, or carer, tends to speak to it in monologues, ie, long stretches of talk that require little feedback or involvement from the child other than its continued attention. From about 1;06 years of age the child is addressed in a grammatically simple manner about a very restricted number of topics. The topics are typically limited to here-and-now concrete concepts, for example, talking about what the child is currently doing or looking at.

From about 2;00 years, words and phrases are repeated to the child over and over again; the mother never seems to say something just once. Moreover, an exaggerated intonation pattern is used, together with a higher than normal pitch. Finally, it also appears that babies attend to a female voice better than to a male voice. Interestingly, there was an attempt to exploit this finding several years ago, by teaching foreign languages by having students listen solely to tapes of female speakers rather than males. An argument against the necessity of motherese is that certain studies have shown that children appear to learn language just as well when their primary carers do not use motherese when speaking to them. Also, it has been suggested that we have underestimated how much language learning occurs through children listening to other adults conversing with each other rather than through their own direct interaction with adults.

Performance and Competence
We have seen that innatists argue that human beings have an innate ability to understand the grammar of languages, that the general rules of language are internalised within the human brain. As a consequence, people are automatically able to recognise and reject ungrammatical utterances. For example, we would be able to reject the following as ungrammatical, even if we are unable to explain why this is so:

rather boxiness stood heavily coat the fell

For most of us, the ability to communicate using language through the medium of speech comes quite naturally. We just seem to acquire the necessary skills with little conscious effort on our part. Without knowing, we develop many subconscious insights into the nature of human communication. We are able to use these so-called psycholinguistic insights to make judgements and predictions about communication. Take a look at the following pictures (adapted from Berko, 1958) and complete the final statement:

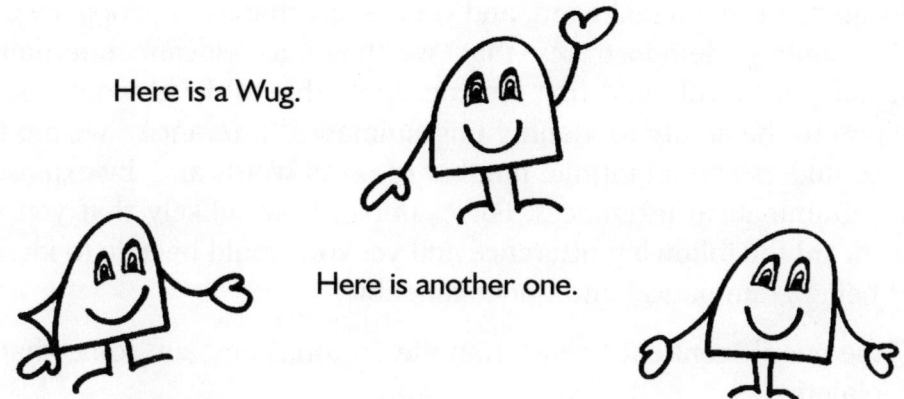

Here is a Wug.

Here is another one.

There are two of them. Now there are two . . .?

If you have understood and internalised the rule that governs how plurals are produced in English, you should have said *Wugs* when completing the statement. It is unlikely that you have come across a real object called a *Wug* before, so you cannot possibly have just memorised this plural form. You have, however, demonstrated that you can apply an internalised psycholinguistic rule to a novel word. You will not only have internalised a rule for the formation of plurals, however. Consider the following:

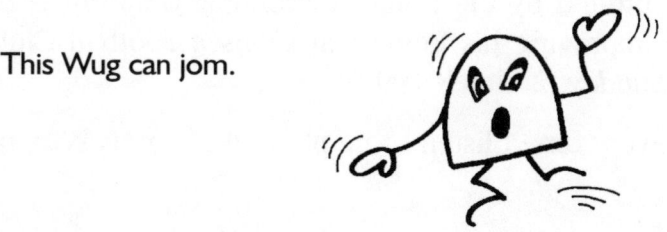

This Wug can jom.

It can't come out to play because it's too busy . . .?

Did you say *jomming*? Most people do. But why not *joms*, or *jomed*, or *rejom*? Well, this is because you have an internalised rule that explains how to create words that describe ongoing actions (what is known as the present progressive). In English this is commonly achieved by the addition of *-ing* to a word. Like the word *Wug* the action word *jom* is fabricated, it is not a real word, and yet the fact that most people respond with *jomming* demonstrates that we have a relevant internalised psycholinguistic rule and that we can apply this to novel words. So, in addition to the ability to identify ungrammatical utterances, we are also able to understand an infinite number of novel words and, by extension, novel grammatical utterances. For example, it is unlikely that you will have heard the following utterance and yet you would be able to identify it as being grammatical and understandable:

the puerile sentient beings from the Truton sphere are somewhat plaintive

This ability to make use of an internalised grammar, which enables us to both speak and understand an infinite number of potential utterances, is known as a speaker's competence. It is competence in the use of language that makes possible a speaker's performance, ie, the behaviour of producing actual utterances. In broad terms, competence may be viewed as an abstract, internalised ability, whereas performance is the behaviour of producing concrete utterances. In essence, it is the difference between what is potential and what is actual. An obvious disparity between competence and performance is the case of foreigners attempting to speak a language other than their first language. Consider the following uttered by the Italian soccer star Gianfranco Zola on the difficulties of improving his English at Chelsea Football Club, England (*The Mail on Sunday*, 2 March 1997):

I try but every time I listen some place like Dennis Wise my English go down

As we know that Zola can speak fluent Italian, we can be confident that he has language competency. However, his performance in a language other than his native Italian does not meet the criteria that most native speakers of English would consider necessary for an utterance to be viewed as grammatical. However, even among native speakers of English there is disagreement about what is considered to be grammatical and what is not. This issue will be touched upon in succeeding chapters.

Early Language Development

Recall that linguistic ability is the ability to manipulate symbols – specifically the arbitrary symbols that we call words – in order to create meaning. The developing child does not, of course, acquire this ability all at once. There are several stages, each incorporating different behaviours, that may be seen as precursors to the acquisition of full linguistic ability. These stages are typically divided into two categories: pre-linguistic (or pre-symbolic) development and linguistic development.

Pre-Linguistic Development

As linguistic development designates the stage when children are able to manipulate verbal symbols, it should be apparent that pre-linguistic development refers to the stage before the child is able to manipulate such symbols. Pre-linguistic development, therefore, concerns itself with precursors to the development of symbolic skills, such as (1) reflexive crying and vegetative sounds, (2) cooing and laughter, (3) vocal play, and (4) babbling (Stark, 1986). This subsection outlines each of these four stages from birth to around 1;01 years of age.

Reflexive Crying and Vegetative Sounds (0–0;02 years)
The sounds used in this stage are the natural sounds that babies make, for example, crying, coughing, burping, swallowing. These sounds have no real communicative significance: the baby cries reflexively because it is hungry or uncomfortable; it burps because it has wind, and so on.

Cooing and Laughter (0;02–0;05 years)
These vocalisations usually occur when the baby is comfortable and content. They are typically made up of vowel and consonant sounds.

Vocal Play (0;04–0;08 years)
At this stage the infant engages in longer and more continuous streams of either vowel or consonant sounds.

Babbling (0;06–1;01 years)
This is the stage most commonly thought of as being associated with language development. It is the stage through which most parents

remember their child passing. It is often, however, regarded as consisting of two sub-stages. The first is reduplicated babbling, in which the child produces a series of consonant-vowel (CV) syllables with the same consonant being repeated, for example:

wa-wa-wa
ab-ab-ab
mu-mu-mu

The second sub-stage is non-reduplicated babbling. This consists of vocalisations either in the form of consonant-vowel-consonant (CVC) sequences, for exampleL

bob
mam
pip

or vowel-consonant-vowel (VCV) sequences, for exampleL

obo
ama
ipi

Up to this stage of development much of what the child produces is really no more than a sort of verbal play. The child is practising individual sounds, and sound sequences, and gaining the motor skills necessary to produce what will eventually be considered as actual adult words. It is this emergence of words that signals the onset of linguistic development.

Linguistic Development
Linguistic development occurs at what is called the One Word Stage (see Blom, 1973; Knowles & Masidlover, 1982; Harris, 1990). It is at this stage that we can talk properly about a child's expressive language, that is, the words used to express emotions, feelings, wants, needs, ideas, and so on. This should not be confused with the child's understanding or receptive language. The two are, of course, closely related. However, children will typically understand much more than they can actually express and a

child's expressive language, therefore, lags behind its comprehension by a few months.

Early One Word Stage (1;00–1;07 years)
Before the emergence of the first 'adult' words the child will use specific sound combinations in particular situations. The sound combinations are not conventional adult words, but they appear to be being used consistently to express meaning. For example, if the child says *mu* every time it is offered a bottle of milk then this may be considered to be a 'real' word. Similarly, if the child says *bibi* each time it is given a biscuit then, even though the sound combination does not represent an exact adult word, it would still be considered an early word. These early words are called 'protowords'. The child will also be using gesture together with these specific vocalisations in order to obtain needs, express emotions, and so on. The important point is that the child is consistent in its use of a particular 'word'.

Later One Word Stage (1;02–2;00 years)
The words used by the child are now more readily identifiable as actual adult words. A variety of single words are used to express its feelings, needs, wants, and so on. This is the stage at which, among other things, the child begins to name and label the objects and people around it. Examples include common nouns such as:

cup
dog
hat

proper nouns such as:

Dad
Sarah
Rover

and verbs such as:

kiss
go
sit.

The child may also use a few social words such as:

no
bye-bye
please

The child will not yet have developed all the adult speech sounds, and so the words used are unlikely to sound exactly as an adult would say them. However, they are beginning to approximate more closely to an adult model and they are beginning to be used consistently. At the end of the One Word Stage the child should have a much larger vocabulary, be able to sustain a simple conversation, use several adult speech sounds appropriately and convey meaning through the use of single words in combination with facial expression, gesture and actions. These single words will express a variety of meaning. The next stage in the child's development of expressive language is that it begins to combine two words into simple phrases.

Two Word Stage (1;08–2;06 years)
It is at this stage that the child begins to produce two-word combinations similar to the following:

daddy car
shoe on
where Katie

Note that a variety of different word classes may be combined. For example, *daddy car* involves the combination of one noun (*daddy*) with another noun (*car*). However, *shoe on* consists of a noun (*shoe*) plus a preposition (*on*). Also, *where Katie* uses an interrogative pronoun (*where*) together with a proper noun (*Katie*). In fact, a high percentage of these two-word combinations incorporate nouns. This is not surprising, as the child has spent a lot of time learning the names of objects and people. These are the important things in its environment and the things that are most likely to be manipulated, talked about, and so on. They are the concrete, permanent things to which the child can most readily relate. In addition, at this Two Word Stage there is also prolific use of verbs.

Three Word Stage (2;04–3;06 years)
As its name implies, at this next stage of developme
their two-word utterances by incorporating at least a...
reality children may add up to two more words, thereby creati...
utterances as long as four words. The child makes greater use of pronouns
at this stage, for example:

> *me* kiss mummy
> *you* make toy
> *he* hit ball

It is at this stage that the child also begins to use the articles *the*, *a*
and *an*. At first their use is inconsistent, but as the child approaches 3;06
years they become more consolidated in their utterances, for example:

> me kick *a* ball
> you give *the* dolly
> he hit *the* ball

In addition, it is common for the prepositions *in* and *on* to be
incorporated between two nouns or pronouns, for example:

> mummy *on* bed
> you *in* it
> Sarah *in* bath

Four Word Stage (2;10–4;00 years)
From about 2;10 years the child begins to combine between four and six
words in any one utterance. There is greater use of contrast between
prepositions such as *in*, *on* and *under* and adjectives such as *big* and *little*,
for example:

> mummy on *little* bed
> daddy under *big* car
> daddy playing with the *little* ball

Complex Utterance Stage (4;00–5;00 years)
This stage is typified by longer utterances, with the child regularly
producing utterances of over six words in length. It is at this stage that the

concept of past and future time develops, and this is expressed linguistically in a child's utterances, for example:

we all went to see Ryan *yesterday*   [past time]
Daddy *is going to get* a shoe   [future time]
Robert *stopped* and *kicked* a good goal   [past time]

Some of the more conceptually difficult prepositions such as *behind*, *in front* and *next to* also become established at this stage. The child will also be using the contracted negative, that is, *can't* rather than *can not*, *didn't* rather than *did not*, *won't* rather than *will not*, and so on. Example utterances include the following:

Helen *can't* go to granddad's house
Connor *didn't* stop crying
he *won't* eat up all his dinner for mummy

There is a lot of controversy about just when the Complex Utterance Stage is completed. Some researchers claim that at 5;00 years of age a child has developed all of the major adult linguistic features, and that the only real progression beyond this stage is the further acquisition of vocabulary items. Other researchers, however, argue that children up to the age of 12;00 years are still developing adult syntax (see McTear, 1985; Crystal, 1986).

As indicated, our overview of language development has focused on how the child develops longer and longer utterances, that is, we have concentrated on expressive language. It should be noted, however, that there is a parallel development of comprehension, or receptive language. So, for example, at the early One Word Stage the child is capable of understanding a few single words spoken by others as well as speaking a few words. Similarly, at the Three Word Stage the child can also comprehend the four- to six-word utterances spoken by others as well as producing such utterances itself. In summary, the child will need to be able to comprehend utterances at least at the same level as those that it is able to construct and use expressively. In reality, we find that a child's level of understanding actually precedes its level of expression. That is to say, a normally developing child will always understand more than it can express. The extent to which the development of receptive language precedes expressive language is highly variable, and it is not possible to define any precise norms in relation to this. Table 2.1 summarises the stages of early development of expressive language.

Table 2.1 *Early Development of Expressive Language*

Precursors to Language (Pre-Linguistic)

0–0;02 years	0;02–0;05 years	0;04–0;08 years	0;06–1;01 years
reflexive crying and vegetative sounds	cooing and laughter	vocal play	babbling – reduplicated – non-reduplicated

(Symbolic) Language

1;00–1;07 years	1;02–2;00 years	1;08–2;06 years
Early One Word Stage – protowords	Later One Word Stage	Two Word Stage

2;04–3;06 years	2;10–4;00 years	4;00–5;00 years
Three Word Stage	Four Word Stage	Complex Utterance Stage

Mean Length of Utterance (MLU)

From the foregoing discussion of pre-linguistic and linguistic development, two points can be made. First, as children mature the length of their utterances increases and, second, all children appear to develop expressive language in the same sequential order. Consequently we are able to relate the length of an utterance to a child's age. Thus, we can say that at 1;08–2;06 years of age utterances are typically two words long; at 2;04–3;06 years they are up to four words long; at 2;10–4;00 years they are up to six words long; and from 4;00 years they are usually longer than six words. It should be possible, therefore, to measure the typical length of a child's utterances and determine whether or not this is in keeping with what would be expected for the age of the child. Clearly, it is not sufficient to examine just one utterance, as there is a great deal of variation in the length of utterances. If I ask you, 'Where do you live?' you could answer simply, 'Hull', or 'In Hull', or 'I live in Hull', and so on.

It is necessary, therefore, to examine several utterances and then to calculate the average length of utterance based on a count of the number of individual words[1] in each utterance. We will now provide an example of how to calculate a mean length of utterance (MLU).

Suppose we have heard a 4;00-year-old child produce the following utterances:

> go home now
> I live in Billingham
> mummy kiss my nice daddy
> I like your dog
> what a nice blue car

We can calculate the MLU as follows. Taking each utterance in turn, we count the number of words in the utterances. So, we would analyse the utterances as follows:

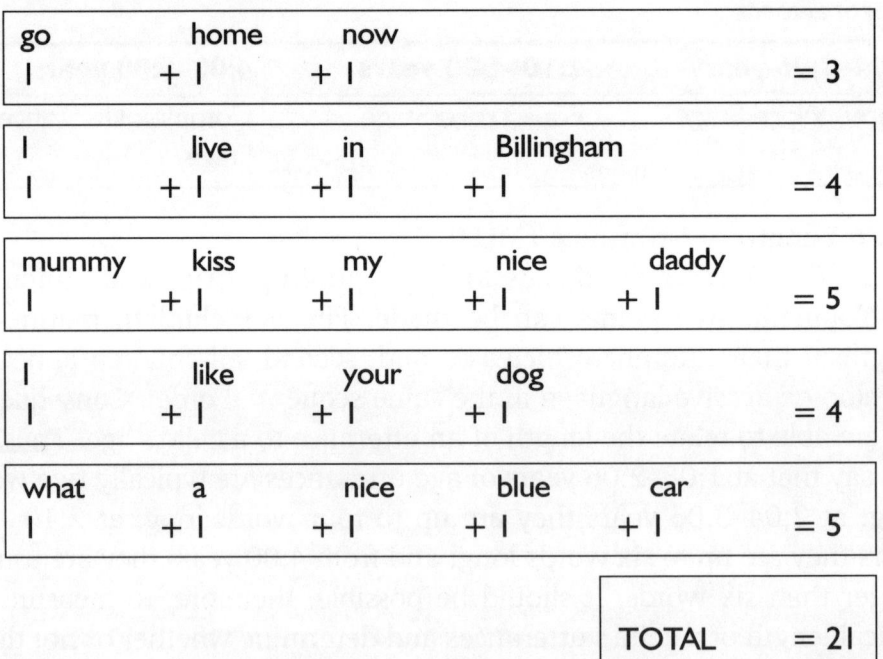

go	home	now			
I	+ I	+ I			= 3

I	live	in	Billingham		
I	+ I	+ I	+ I		= 4

mummy	kiss	my	nice	daddy	
I	+ I	+ I	+ I	+ I	= 5

I	like	your	dog		
I	+ I	+ I	+ I		= 4

what	a	nice	blue	car	
I	+ I	+ I	+ I	+ I	= 5

TOTAL	= 21

Therefore there is a total of 21 words. Now, in order to find the mean length of utterance we take the total number of words (21) and divide it by the total number of utterances (5). Thus, the mean length of utterance is 21/5 = 4.20. What we need to do now is determine the age at which the majority of children would present with a mean length of utterance equivalent to the one our particular child has scored. This is known as the age equivalent. We do this by reading off the age equivalent from Table 2.2. From the table, we see that an MLU of 4.20 lies between 4.09 and 4.40. We can conclude, therefore, that an MLU of 4.20 would be expected in a child of between 3;09 and 4;00 years of age. As we know that our particular child is 4;00 years old, then it appears that the average length of the child's utterances is age-appropriate. This suggests, therefore, that this child's language skills are developing along normal lines.

Table 2.2 *Mean Length of Utterance (MLU) by Age*

MLU	age equivalent in years (within 1 month)
1.31	1;06
1.62	1;09
1.92	2;00
2.54	2;06
2.85	2;09
3.16	3;00
3.47	3;03
3.78	3;06
4.09	3;09
4.40	4;00
4.71	4;03
5.02	4;06
5.32	4;09
5.63	5;00

Source: Miller, 1981

A final note on calculating an MLU is worth making. While an analysis of five utterances is better than analysing just one (we would have an MLU of 3.00 if we had analysed only the child's first utterance *go home now*), five utterances is still not enough to achieve any degree of accuracy. Ideally one should analyse no fewer than 50 utterances. Clearly, the more utterances that can be analysed then the more accurate will be the result.

In the next chapter we begin an examination of the building blocks of language: words. We will see how words themselves are composed of smaller elements and how words may be classified according to their function.

Revision Exercises

2.1 List five key properties of language.

2.2 Which develops first, *langage* or *langue*? Explain.

2.3 Which of the following pairs of words collocate highly?

> *knife/fork*
> *concrete/window*
> *cup/spoon*
> *cat/key*
> *black/coffee*

2.4 Calculate a mean length of utterance (MLU) for a 3;04-year-old child who was heard to say the following:

> *I like cheese*
> *my mum play*
> *where daddy*
> *kick ball*
> *Harry*
> *see my mum play ball*

Is this MLU age-appropriate?

Activities

2.5 Observe an adult talking to a pre-linguistic child (ie, below 1;00 years of age), and list the ways in which the adult's speech and language appears to differ from that used when speaking to another adult.

2.6 Observe a young child of between 0;04 and 0;08 years of age and make a list of the speech sounds that the child uses. List any examples of reduplicated and non-reduplicated babbling. Are these CV, CVC or VCV?

2.7 Observe a 3-year-old child playing and talking with another child. Record at least 50 examples of the child's utterances. Analyse the length of these utterances and determine what linguistic stage of development the child has attained. Does this correlate with what you would expect of a child this age? If not, can you explain the discrepancy?

Note

1   *A more accurate measure of the length of an utterance is obtained not by counting words, but by counting what are known as morphemes. These are the various elements from which a word is constructed, such as prefixes and suffixes. Table 2.2 presents figures for a mean length of utterance based on morpheme count. For now, however, it will serve our purpose to count utterance length in words. Morphemes will be discussed in the next chapter.*

CHAPTER 3
Building Words

W E NOTED IN THE PREVIOUS CHAPTER that language has two levels of organisation, a property known as duality. This means that units at the primary level are composed of elements at the secondary level. In this chapter we consider the concept of duality and examine how secondary elements compose the primary units, ie, words. First, we describe the smallest element in a language capable of expressing meaning. This is the morpheme. We then demonstrate how prefixes and suffixes can be added to a free morpheme in order to alter its meaning, and we highlight the difference between free and bound morphemes. Next we consider the primary level of organisation. Nine word classes are recognised: verbs, nouns, adjectives, adverbs, numerals, determiners, pronouns, prepositions and conjunctions. Each word class is seen to incorporate words that all perform a similar function. First, a distinction is made between open and closed word classes – that is, those that can be expanded and those that cannot – and then each class is outlined in turn.

The Morpheme
We have noted that language is a set of symbols used to transmit meaning. But just what is the smallest element of meaning in a language? Most people tend to think of a word as being the smallest element. Is this the case? Consider the following words:

dog	dogs
walk	walked
sad	sadly
run	running

If you were to look up these words in a dictionary you would not find them listed as eight separate words. You would find only four listings of the words in the first column, ie, *dog, walk, sad* and *run*. The words in the second column would be shown within each listing as a variation of the listed word. For example, the word *dog* is used to mean a domesticated animal belonging to the same family as the fox, wolf and jackal. The word *dogs* would then be shown as the plural of *dog*, ie, meaning more than one. Grammatically, then, words can be divided into smaller elements. In the example just discussed, one such element is *dog* and the other element is *-s*, which can be added to *dog* to make it plural. These smaller elements are known as morphemes. There are many other examples of the morpheme *-s* being added to other morphemes to make them plural. Some examples include:

cat-s
hat-s
rat-s

With the earlier example of *walk* and *walked*, the morpheme *-ed* is used to indicate the past tense, ie, that something happened before the present time. Other examples include:

thank-ed
work-ed
pray-ed

The example of *sad* and *sadly* indicates how the morpheme *-ly* has been added to the morpheme *sad* to produce an adverb, ie, a word which indicates how an action was performed. Other examples include:

loud-ly
proud-ly
sincere-ly

The final example of *run* and *running* indicates how the morpheme *-ing* has been added to the morpheme *run* to denote an ongoing action. Further examples are:

sitt-ing
ring-ing
sing-ing

You will have noticed that, in some instances, when a morpheme is added to another morpheme the spelling of the morpheme which has been added to changes. This is true of *run* → *running* (where an extra *n* is inserted), *sit* → *sitting* (where an extra *t* is inserted). In the case of *smile* → *smiling*, the *e* of *smile* is omitted, and with *funny* → *funnily*, the *y* of *funny* is replaced with an *i*. These structural changes in the way we write the word do not alter the meaning that is produced by the combination of the morphemes.

So far, all the cited examples have involved adding morphemes to the ends of other morphemes. Morphemes in this position are known as suffixes. Morphemes could, of course, be added to the front of other morphemes, in which case they are known as prefixes. Examples of this are *re-* as in *reprint, repaint* and *redo*; *pre-* as in *preordain, prepay* and *prefix*, and *dis-* as in *disallow, disarm* and *disagree*. It is also possible to alter the meaning of morphemes by the combined use of both prefixes and suffixes. Consider how the morpheme *organise* might be altered below:

Add prefixes and suffixes to the following word to create new meanings:
(prefixes)   organise   (suffixes)

Possible new meanings may be created as follows:

re-	organise	-ed
dis-		-er
		-ation
		-ing
		-s

Bound and Free Morphemes

It should be apparent from the above discussion that some morphemes can occur solely on their own and still convey meaning. Examples of such so-called free morphemes are *go, stop, sit, bus, like* and *organise* (as in the above example). Some types of morpheme, however, cannot occur on their own, eg, *-ly, -ing, -ed, -er, -s, dis-, re-*. These morphemes must always be bound to another morpheme if they are to be meaningful. Consequently, these morphemes are said to be bound morphemes. You will also notice from the above example of how *organise* may be altered that *organise* is the central morpheme. It is this so-called root morpheme which is altered by the addition of the affixes *re-* and *dis-* (prefixes) and *-ed, -er, -ation, -ing* and *-s* (suffixes). For most English words the root is usually a word in its own right and it is typically a free morpheme. There are, however, examples of root morphemes that are not free. An example of such a bound root occurs in the word *unconscionable*, where *un-* can be related to the *un-* of *unrelate, unjustified, unlawful* and so on. However, *conscionable* cannot occur on its own, it always appears bound to the prefix *un-*. Another example is *precocious*, where *pre-* may be associated with the *pre-* in *prenatal, premature, prearrange*, and so on, but, again, *cocious* only appears bound with this prefix. A third example is the word *dissuade*. Here, the prefix *dis-* can be related to the *dis-* of *disagree, disappear* and *dislike* but *suade* cannot appear on its own. A final example is *rescind*, where *re-* equates with the *re-* in words such as *reroute, re-engage* and *reconsider* but *scind* cannot occur on its own. Having introduced the concept of the morpheme we will now turn our attention to a consideration of word classes.

Open and Closed Word Classes

All free morphemes are derived from what are known as word classes. Each word class incorporates words that all perform a similar function. In English, we recognise nine word classes: (1) verbs, (2) nouns, (3) adjectives, (4) adverbs, (5) numerals, (6) determiners, (7) pronouns, (8) prepositions, and (9) conjunctions. In addition, each word class is considered to be either 'open' or 'closed'. The four English word classes of verbs, nouns, adjectives and adverbs constitute the open classes. This is because, in principle, there is no upper limit to the number of words that can be entered into the class. As language changes over time new words are constantly being added. Relatively new words that have been added to the word class of verbs are *hoover* as in *I've just hoovered the carpet* (meaning, 'I have just cleaned the carpet with a vacuum cleaner') and *xerox* as in *Can you xerox this for me?* (meaning, 'Can you photocopy this for me?'). New words can only be added to the open word classes. The remaining five word classes – numerals, determiners, pronouns, prepositions and conjunctions – have a fixed number of words that perform a similar function. No new words can be added to these classes. For example, in the utterance *I have a ball* the word *I* is a pronoun that refers to the speaker. It is not possible to introduce any new words to substitute for this pronoun. There is no other acceptable way in English to refer to the speaker in this context other than by the use of *I*. Because these word classes cannot be added to, they are referred to as closed classes. We will now consider each word class in turn.

Verbs

Verbs are commonly used to describe actions that are performed by an agent's act of will. Consider the following utterances:

> Margaret *started* her studies last year
> the dog *walked* to its kennel
> I *write* with a pen

In the first example, we see that the action of starting her studies was instigated by Margaret: by exerting independent will she performed an action. In the second example, the dog is the agent that instigates the action of walking and, in the third example, it is *I* who wilfully performs the action of writing. As well as expressing this idea of action, verbs are also capable of expressing other concepts (see chapter 1 of Jackson, 1990). For example, they are used to describe events that happen. Consider the following:

the sick child *improved*

In this utterance, unlike action verbs, there is no explicit reference to an instigator of the event. The event just happened. Consider the following further example:

the ball *hit* the net

Again, there is no stated instigator of the event of the ball hitting the net. Of course, we may speculate that some wilful agent had kicked the ball and that this had caused it to hit the net. However, we are concerned here with an examination of the linguistic utterance, we are not speculating on hypothetical utterances. To reiterate, in the utterances *the sick child improved* and *the ball hit the net*, there is no stated instigator of the event. In fact, this is the main distinguishing feature between action verbs and event verbs – ie, that the former have a stated instigator, while the latter do not. Here are three further examples of event verbs:

the water *boiled*
the lamp *illuminated* the darkness
the ship *landed* in the New World

Finally, verbs are also used to refer to the state of people or things, ie, the way they are, their inner psychological perception or awareness, what condition they are in, and so on. Consider the following:

this cheese *is* awful

The verb *is* tells us something about the state that the cheese is in. Specifically, it describes a quality of the cheese, that it is awful. Now consider the following example:

Kathryn *likes* music

In this utterance, the verb *likes* again indicates a state. On this occasion, it is Kathryn's private, emotional state. It describes something about her inner psychological state, that she expressly likes music. State verbs can, therefore, describe a variety of states of both people and things, including the quality of something and someone's psychological state. Here are a few more examples of state verbs:

I *ache* all down my arm   [describes a private, bodily sensation]
I *believe* we know each other   [describes a private, intellectual state]
a tomato *is* technically a fruit   [describes a quality]

In summary, the words within the word class of verbs function to describe actions, events or states. The largest group of verbs is known as the lexical verbs. These are described in further detail below.

Lexical Verbs
Lexical verbs are the main verbs that are typically cited in a dictionary, ie, they appear in the lexicon. As we have seen, they are the words that describe actions, events and states, for example:

Ven *pulled* the safety belt   [action]
the plums *ripened* on the tree   [event]
Dr Livingstone, I *presume*   [state]

In English there are six discrete forms of almost every lexical verb, irrespective of whether or not they are describing an action, event or state. The verb forms are set out in Table 3.1.

Table 3.1 *English Verb Forms*

no	verb form		examples	
1	PRESENT	*walk*	*push*	*sing*
2	PRESENT (third person singular)	*walks*	*pushes*	*sings*
3	PRESENT PARTICIPLE	*walking*	*pushing*	*singing*
4	PAST	*walked*	*pushed*	*sang*
5	PAST PARTICIPLE	*walked*	*pushed*	*sung*
6	INFINITIVE	*to walk*	*to push*	*to sing*

An important point to notice in Table 3.1 is that the verb forms mark aspects of time. Numbers 1 to 3 are related to the present moment and numbers 4 and 5 relate to states, events or actions in the past. Verbs, therefore, allow us to make distinctions related to just two aspects of time, the present and the past. We will now consider each of the English verb forms in turn.

Present-Tense Verb Forms
There are three verb forms that describe states, events and actions in the present moment. They are (1) present, (2) third person singular, and (3) present participle.

Present
This verb form is the one that is used as the main listing in dictionaries. It is therefore sometimes known as the citation form, because this is the form that is cited in reference books. Examples of its useage include the following:

I *walk* to the office	I *push* carts for a living	I *sing* in the Friday Choir
you *walk* to the office	you *push* carts for a living	you *sing* in the Friday Choir
we *walk* to the office	we *push* carts for a living	we *sing* in the Friday Choir
they *walk* to the office	they *push* carts for a living	they *sing* in the Friday Choir

Notice that the form of the verb remains the same whether or not the person performing the action is *I, you, we* or *they*.

Third person singular
Now contrast the verb form in the following utterances with those presented immediately above. In these examples, the person carrying out the action is *he, she* or *it*:

he *walks* to the office	he *pushes* carts for a living	he *sings* in the Friday Choir
she *walks* to the office	she *pushes* carts for a living	she *sings* in the Friday Choir
it *walks* to the office	it *pushes* carts for a living	it *sings* in the Friday Choir

Notice, this time, that the verb forms are inflected, that is, an additional morpheme is appended: *walk* becomes *walks*, *push* becomes *pushes* and *sing* becomes *sings*. These verb forms are examples of the second type of present tense in English, the third person singular. It should be apparent, therefore, that a difference between the two verb forms is related to the category of person. As we have seen, person refers to the person or thing performing a particular action. If the person is the speaker then we refer to this as the first person. If the person is the one being addressed then this is the second person. If the person is the one who is being talked about then this is the third person. Each person is associated with different pronouns (these are discussed later in the chapter). The first person is associated with *I* and *we*, the second person with *you*, and the third person with *he, she, it* and *they*. The category of person can then be further subdivided by number. Number refers to whether or not reference is being made to one thing (singular) or more than one thing (plural). You may have noticed that some of the pronouns associated with person are singular (*I, you, he, she, it*), and some are plural (*we, you, they*). Table 3.2 summarises the use of pronouns to mark person and number.

Table 3.2 *Pronouns, Person and Number*

| number | person | | |
	1st	2nd	3rd
singular	*I*	*you*	*he, she, it*
plural	*we*	*you*	*they*

To reiterate, with respect to the verbs *walk*, *push* and *sing*, the forms *walks*, *pushes* and *sings* are associated with the third person singular, while the forms *walk*, *push* and *sing* are associated with all other persons and numbers.

Present participle

There is a third verb form that relates to the present moment. This is the present participle. Like the third person singular verb form, the present participle is also constructed by the addition of a morpheme to the citation form. In this instance, however, it is the morpheme *-ing*. The present participle functions to convey the sense of a person or thing being engaged in a continuing action, for example:

> I am *walking* to Land's End
> he is *pushing* very quickly
> Anya is still *singing*

Past-Tense Verb Forms

In contrast to the three verb forms of the present tense, for almost every verb there are just two verb forms that describe states, events and actions in the past, that is, before the present moment. They are the past, and the past participle.

Past

The majority of English verbs form their past tense by the addition of the morpheme *-ed*, as in the following examples:

> Daniel *walked* to the concert
> the envelopes were *pushed* through the door
> Anya *talked* all evening

Verbs that form their past tense in this manner are referred to as regular verbs, as they follow a regular pattern. However, there are about 300 verbs that do not follow this regular pattern. These form their past tense by a change in the spelling and pronunciation of the word, rather than by the addition of *-ed*. They are therefore known as irregular verbs. The irregular past verb form example shown in Table 3.1 is *sang*. Other examples of irregular verbs and their past tenses include the following:

Irregular verb	Past tense
eat	ate
bring	brought
swing	swung
catch	caught
choose	chose

Past Participle

We noted that the present participle functions to convey the sense of a continuing action in the present moment. In contrast, the past participle functions to convey the sense of a person or thing having undergone an action in the past. For regular verbs the past participle has the same form as the past tense, for example:

she *walked* away	[past]
she had *walked* away	[past participle]
it *pushed* the door	[past]
it has *pushed* the door	[past participle]

For many verbs, however, there is a difference between the past tense form and the past participle form, for example:

she *sang* her last song	[past]
she has *sung* her last song	[past participle]
I *took* the book	[past]
I have *taken* the book	[past participle]

Infinitive

This form of the verb is easily recognised because a *to* typically precedes the citation form. Examples of the use of the infinitive include the following:

Jordan has *to walk* to the shops
I would like *to eat* now
he wants *to go* out

'Future' Tense
We saw in Table 3.1 that English verb forms mark only two aspects of time, the present and the past, there is no future tense form of English verbs. Some languages do mark future tense with a particular verb form, however. French is one such language, for example, 'je mangerai' (*I will eat*), 'tu danseras' (*you will dance*) 'ils donneront' (*they will give*). Speakers of English are, however, clearly capable of speaking not only in terms of the past and the present but also in terms of the future. How then do we indicate future time in English? There are four main ways: the use of (1) temporal markers, (2) *will/shall*, (3) *be going to*, and (4) *be about to*. We will consider each of these in turn.

Temporal markers
One of the most obvious ways of referring to any moment in time is to use so-called temporal markers. Temporal markers can refer to the past (eg, *yesterday, last Sunday, the other day*), present (eg, *now, at present, currently*) and future (eg, *tomorrow, next week, in a fortnight*). Examples of utterances that use temporal markers to indicate future time include the following:

> when I give it to you *tomorrow*, don't laugh
> Adam is singing *next week*
> I'm leaving *tonight*

Will/shall
The words *will* and *shall* are used in constructions such as the following:

> I *will* send you a postcard
> I *shall* leave you alone
> you *will* never amount to anything

Be going to
Reference to the future can be achieved by using the verb *be* followed by *going to* as in the following examples:

> I *am going to* cut the cake
> you *are going to* have a nice time
> she *is going to* visit the Louvre

Be about to

Again, reference to the future can be made through the use of the verb *be* but, this time, followed by *about to*. Consider the following examples:

>he *is about to* release the capsule
>they *are about to* free the prisoners
>we *are about to* confess it all

Auxiliary Verbs

Before closing our discussion of verbs, there is one further subdivision that needs to be highlighted. As well as the enormous number of lexical verbs, there is a limited number of so-called auxiliary verbs. These have a mainly grammatical function. We have already met some of them when we considered the present and past participles. Consider the following example of the use of a present participle:

>the boy *is* crying

In this utterance the word *crying* is considered to be the lexical verb. Its citation form would, of course, be *cry*. But consider the word *is*. We know that this is a verb, as it is derived from the verb *be* or *to be*. In this context, however, the word does not appear to convey any specific meaning of its own. It appears to have a largely grammatical function, serving to signal the present participle in its association with the *-ing* morpheme. The word *is* in this context is not, therefore, a lexical verb but it is described as an auxiliary verb. There are two types of auxiliary verb: primary auxiliaries and modal auxiliaries.

Primary auxiliaries

The main primary auxiliary verbs are *be* and *have*, for example:

be:	I *am* going
	he *is* singing
	she *was* writing
have:	I *have* gone
	he *has* sung
	she *has* written

Modal auxiliaries

These indicate the mood or attitude of the speaker and include items such as *can*, *could*, *should*, *must* and *may*, for example:

> I *may* go
> he *should* sing
> she *can* write

This completes our discussion of verbs. We now turn our attention to the largest open word class, nouns.

Nouns

As indicated, nouns compose by far the largest class of words. This is because they are generally used to name things. As there is an almost infinite number of things to be named the class is expansive. In addition, as humankind progresses and discovers new things, so we need new words to describe the things we have discovered. Therefore this class is constantly being added to. Recent new nouns in English include *mobile* as in *I will be on my mobile* (meaning, 'I will be using my portable telephone if you need to contact me') and *fax* as in *Send me a fax tomorrow* (meaning, 'Send me an electronically transmitted facsimile of the document tomorrow'). Societies tend to name those things that are important to them, a process known as nominalisation. Thus, it is not unusual that many of the new nouns describe objects that are technological advancements. In comparison, most Europeans are likely to use only the one word for *snow*. This is because it is largely unimportant for most of these peoples because the climate is not predominantly sub-arctic. In the languages spoken by the Inuit peoples of North America, however, there are up to 20 words for snow, each word reflecting a difference that the Inuit peoples perceive in the various types of snow within the environment they inhabit. Snow is, clearly, a more important object to these peoples than to most Europeans. Nouns can be divided into two broad contrasting categories: proper nouns and common nouns. These are described below.

Proper Nouns

These nouns refer to unique things, people, places, institutions, and so on, for example:

Tower of London	[thing]
Adam	[person]
Newcastle	[place]
Department of Health	[institution]

Common Nouns
These refer to a category of objects or to a specific instance of that category, for example:

Category	**S**pecific instance
trees	tree
animals	animal
cups	cup

Nouns can be further subdivided into concrete nouns and abstract nouns, as follows:

Concrete Nouns
These nouns refer to perceivable, tangible objects in the world, for example:

    cup
    book
    house

Abstract Nouns
These refer to things that are intangible, such as ideas and emotions, for example:

    happiness
    love
    friendship

A third subdivision involves the notion of quantity and separates the nouns into countable nouns and mass nouns.

Countable Nouns
These nouns represent objects that can be counted. This implies, therefore, that it is possible to have more than one of the object in question, for example:

cat	[*five cats*]
computer	[*two computers*]
brother	[*three brothers*]

Mass Nouns
These nouns contrast with countable nouns in that they are uncountable. Examples include:

water
flour
hay

It is not generally possible to have, for example, *two waters, three flours* or *four hays*, and so on.

Therefore we can, describe every noun in the English language in terms of the above three contrastive categories, that is, (1) common/proper, (2) concrete/abstract, and (3) countable/mass. For example, the word *table* would be described as a common, concrete, countable noun, whereas the word *love* is a common, abstract, mass noun. Nouns can be represented diagrammatically, as in Table 3.3.

Table 3.3 *Classification of Nouns*

noun	common	proper	concrete	abstract	countable	mass
table	✔		✔		✔	
love	✔			✔		✔
John		✔	✔		✔	
Sterling		✔	✔			✔
tension	✔			✔		✔

Note that while the word *tension* has been described in Table 3.3 as a mass noun, on the basis that one would not generally talk of 'two tensions', 'three tensions', and so on, it is possible to postulate an occasion in which the noun could be described as countable. Consider the following:

there are three *tensions* in the political arena

On this occasion, the noun *tension* is in plural form because there is an implicit reference to an ability to actually count tensions (eg, those from the far-right, the centre-left and the far-left of the political arena). The same sort of argument could be assumed for the words *flour* and *hay*, which we defined earlier as mass nouns. For example, if you were thinking of different strains of flour or types of hay, you might be able to construct meaningful utterances such as:

we are considering the three types of *flours* available to bakers
the farmer is sorting the four types of *hays* into separate barns

Thus, the description and meanings assigned to words are dependent upon their context of occurrence. This issue is considered in Chapter 5, where we examine the notion of semantics. We will now investigate the third open class of English words, adjectives.

Adjectives
Adjectives are descriptors that qualify nouns by providing additional and specific information. They may be used in a variety of ways, but the two most common are: before a noun and the use of the copula.

Before a Noun
Adjectives frequently occur immediately before a noun in English, as in the following example:

	Adjective	**Noun**
the	*small*	house

In this utterance, we can see that the adjective *small* qualifies the noun that it precedes. In other words, it provides a more specific description of the following noun. We now know what sort of house is being referred to, ie, it is a *small* house. The adjective, therefore, qualifies the noun *house*. It provides additional descriptive information that explains more fully the sort of house that is being referred to. We are able to infer that the house is not a big house because the additional information provided by the adjective indicates that it is a *small* house. Consider the next example:

	Adjective	**Noun**
Helen's	*happy*	brother

Again, we see that the adjective precedes the noun. Once more, it serves to qualify this noun. In particular, it tells us something about Helen's brother's emotional state. We now realise that Helen's brother is *happy*. In summary, adjectives provide additional descriptive information by qualifying nouns. The nouns may be qualified in a variety of ways. For example, an adjective may tell us something about the shape of an object (*round, square, flat*), its size (*big, small, tiny*), its colour (*red, yellow, blue*), its emotional state (*happy, sad, anxious*), its physical condition (*cold, hot, wet*), its position (*left, right, central*) and so on. Here are a few more examples:

	Adjective	**Noun**	
your	*square*	box	[shape]
the	*small*	house	[size]
Eric's	*red*	shirt	[colour]
the	*upset*	child	[emotional state]
the	*soggy*	pitch	[condition]
my	*left*	foot	[position]

Use of the Copula

As well as occurring immediately before a noun, adjectives may also be joined to a noun by what is known as a copula. This is the use of verbs like *be* or *become* to join, or couple, the noun to the adjective. Consider the following example:

Noun	**Copula**	**Adjective**
Kathryn	is	*lovely*

In this utterance, the adjective appears at the end but serves to provide additional descriptive information about the preceding noun *Kathryn*. The noun and the adjective are coupled together through the use of the copula *is*, derived from the verb *be*. So we now understand something more about the kind of person Kathryn is, ie, that she is *lovely*. Other examples of adjectives combined with nouns by the copula are as follows:

	Noun	Copula	Adjective
his	girlfriend	became	*upset*
the	supporters	are	*ecstatic*
Sam's	mother	is	*overjoyed*

This completes our discussion of adjectives and we now turn our attention to the fourth, and final, open word class in English, adverbs.

Adverbs

Adverbs are words that are used to modify a verb, adjective or another adverb. They are typically used to provide circumstantial information such as the time, place, manner, degree, cause, etc, of an action or event. Adverbs can often be left out of utterances without making them nonsensical, as they often provide gratuitous information that is not essential for understanding. Consider the following utterance:

John painted the picture *quickly*

The adverb *quickly* functions to describe the manner in which John painted the picture. This information is said to be gratuitous because if it is omitted (ie, *John painted the picture*) we can still understand the essential meaning, that John painted a picture. Similarly, in the following utterance, the adverb *yesterday* can be omitted without spoiling the essential meaning:

the therapists ate at Rossi's *yesterday*

By omitting the adverb *yesterday* we still understand that the therapists ate at Rossi's. Of course, adverbs do provide additional meaning, in this case we now understand something more about the actual time when the therapists ate. This is an example of a temporal adverb. There are four main types of adverb: (1) temporal, (2) locative, (3) manner, and (4) intensifying. Each of these will be described below.

Temporal Adverbs

Temporal adverbs are used to specify the timing of an action or event. For example:

she went home *yesterday*
the team won the competition *last weekend*
next week we will visit Hartlepool

Locative Adverbs

These adverbs supply information related to the location of an event or action, or the direction of an action. For example:

> Kathy went *outside* to collect her products
> they travelled *east* to Darlington
> she turned the knob *anti-clockwise*

Manner Adverbs

These indicate something about the way in which an action or event is performed. For example:

> the boy ran *slowly* to his mother
> *happily*, she took him in her arms
> she asked *nervously*

Intensifying Adverbs

Consider the following utterance:

> the child is *clever*

This utterance describes the state of a child. Specifically, the adjective *clever* serves to qualify the noun *child* by providing additional information. We know that this child has a certain quality, ie, it is a clever child. Certain adjectives allow us to ask further questions. For example, how clever is the child? There is a sense in which the adjective *clever* can be graded or intensified. Consider the following:

> the child is *very* clever

We now have an answer to our question. The child is not just clever, the child is actually *very* clever! *Very* is an adverb that serves to grade, or intensify, the adjective. It is therefore known as an intensifying adverb. Intensifying adverbs do not just modify adjectives, however. They can also be used to modify other adverbs. Consider the following statement:

> Steve hit the shuttlecock *quickly*

In this statement, the adverb *quickly* is used to tell us something about the manner in which Steve hit the shuttlecock, ie, that he did not hit it slowly but rather that he hit it quickly. As before, we can ask questions of certain adverbs, for example, how quickly did Steve hit the shuttlecock? Again, the answer can be provided by the insertion of an intensifying adverb, as follows:

Steve hit the shuttlecock *very* quickly

On this occasion, therefore, the intensifying adverb *very* has been used to modify not an adjective but another adverb. Following are more examples of the use of intensifying adverbs (note that they always precede the associated adjective or adverb):

the dog was *very* quick	[modifies the adjective *quick*]
she was *extremely* quiet	[modifies the adjective *quiet*]
Kulvinder seemed *more* happy	[modifies the adjective *happy*]
the dog moved *very* quickly	[modifies the adverb *quickly*]
she spoke *extremely* quietly	[modifies the adverb *quietly*]
Kulvinder played *more* happily	[modifies the adverb *happily*]

We have now considered all of the English open word classes. The remaining five word classes (numerals, determiners, pronouns, prepositions and conjunctions) are all closed word classes and they will be discussed in the following sections.

Numerals

Recall that a word class is said to be closed if no more words can be added to the class. While in theory it is possible to keep counting to infinity, in practice there are a limited number of numerals that are used to enable this counting process. Numerals are, therefore, categorised as a closed word class. They are divided into just two types: cardinals and ordinals.

Cardinals

These specify numeric quantity, for example:

one
two
three
four … [and so on]

Example utterances that incorporate cardinals include the following:

> I'll have *two* of those, please
> he ran around the track *four* times
> you've got *one* more chance

Ordinals

These numerals specify the order of items, for example:

> first
> second
> third
> fourth ... [and so on]

The following are examples of their use:

> right, that's the *first* button sewn on
> Steve came *second* in his race
> take down your tree on *twelfth* night

Determiners

Determiners are used to determine what is being referred to in an utterance. There are two types of determiner: identifiers and quantifiers. These two categories are described below.

Identifiers

There are four types of identifier: (1) indefinite article, (2) definite article, (3) possessives, and (4) demonstratives. Examples of each are provided below.

Indefinite article

There are just two morphemes in this category, *a* and *an*, for example:

> Jordan has *a* ball
> *an* apple fell on Isaac's head
> Robert is eating *an* orange

The indefinite article *a* is generally used before words that begin with a consonant (eg, *a* <u>*b*</u>*all*, *a* <u>*s*</u>*ock*, *a* <u>*c*</u>*lock*) whereas the indefinite article *an* is generally used before words that begin with a vowel (eg, *an octopus, an agent, an elf*). (consonants and vowels are discussed at length later, in Chapter 6).

Definite article

There is only one definite article in English, *the*, for example:

> throw me *the* ball
> *the* car is terrific
> he spoke in *the* corridor

The difference between the indefinite and definite articles lies in how specific the article is. The indefinite article is used to refer to one of any number of similar items, eg, *a ball* refers to just any one ball from the many available balls. The definite article, in contrast, is more specific as it clearly indicates a special item, eg, *the ball* identifies the particular ball selected from the many available balls.

Possessives

These identifiers serve to indicate ownership and include *my, your, his, her, its, our* and *their*. They are summarised in terms of person and number in Table 3.4.

Table 3.4 *Possessive Identifiers*

number		person	
	1st	2nd	3rd
singular	*my*	*your*	*his, her, its*
plural	*our*	*your*	*their*

Examples of the use of possessive identifiers include the following:

> it is *my* ball
> where are *your* notes?
> that's *her* car

Demonstratives

There are four demonstrative identifiers: *this, that, these* and *those*. Demonstratives are used to indicate the proximity of items. A proximate item (ie, one that is close by) is referred to by using the demonstrative *this*, eg, *this ball in my hand*. More than one proximate item is referred to using *these*, eg, *these balls in my hand*. A single non-proximate item (ie, one that is not close by) is referred to by using *that*, eg, *that ball over there*. More than one non-proximate item is referred to by using *those*, eg, *those balls over there*. This relationship between distance and number is summarised diagrammatically in Table 3.5.

Table 3.5 *Demonstrative Identifiers*

	proximate	non-proximate
singular	*this*	*that*
plural	*these*	*those*

Here are some examples of the use of demonstratives:

this plant needs watering
it fell on *that* house
these boots were made for walking

Quantifiers

Quantifiers are used to make reference to indefinite quantities, eg, *several, few, a little, many*. Examples include the following:

I have *several* jazz albums
the Chief Executive has *many* complaints to make
a little sympathy always helps

Pronouns

Pronouns are words that substitute for nouns (*pro-noun* meaning *for-noun*), eg, *him, they, hers, yours, who, where*. They are usually only meaningful after a noun has already been mentioned. For example, if I began a conversation with, 'He told me to leave. He said it was important', it would be difficult for the listener to know just exactly who I was talking about. Who is the *he* I am referring to? Is it my uncle? The listener's brother? A stranger? The use of the pronoun *he* without previously using a noun is potentially confusing. The conversation would be more readily understood if it had been phrased as follows: 'Jeff told me to leave. He said it was important.' This time it is obvious who is being referred to and it is clear that the pronoun *he* in the second utterance is referring to the noun *Jeff* in the first utterance. Pronouns can be subdivided into five categories: (1) personal, (2) reflexive, (3) demonstrative, (4) interrogative, and (5) indefinite. Each category is discussed in turn below.

Personal Pronouns
There are three subsets of personal pronouns: (1) subjective, (2) objective, and (3) possessive.

Personal pronouns (subjective)
We met this particular subset of personal pronouns when we considered the present tense form of verbs. These were summarised in relation to person and number in Table 3.2 and they are reproduced in Table 3.6 for clarity.

Table 3.6 *Personal Pronouns (Subjective)*

number		person	
	1st	2nd	3rd
singular	*I*	*you*	*he, she, it*
plural	*we*	*you*	*they*

These pronouns substitute for nouns that are functioning as the subject of an utterance. A subject is the thing, or person, performing a particular action. Consider the following:

Paul kissed Judy

In this utterance, *Paul* is the subject as he is the person performing the particular action of kissing. The noun *Paul* can be substituted with the personal pronoun *he* to give the following:

he kissed Judy

Further examples of personal pronouns substituting for subjects include the following:

it bit the child on the hand
they shone the torches
we encouraged Connor to speak

Personal pronouns (objective)

Table 3.7 *Personal Pronouns (Objective)*

| number | | person | |
	1st	2nd	3rd
singular	*me*	*you*	*him, her, it*
plural	*us*	*you*	*them*

The subset of pronouns shown in Table 3.7 substitute for nouns that are functioning as the object of an utterance. The object is the person or thing undergoing an action. Consider again our earlier example:

Paul kissed *Judy*

The person that has undergone Paul's action of kissing is *Judy*. Therefore the noun *Judy* is the object. A pronoun could now be used to substitute for this noun, as follows:

Paul kissed *her*

Further examples of pronouns substituting for nouns that are functioning as objects include the following:

the dog bit *him*
Bob and Duncan shone *them*
Kathryn, Margaret and I encouraged *him*

Personal pronouns (possessive)

The third subset of personal pronouns is shown in Table 3.8. The title is self-explanatory, ie, they are used to indicate possession of something.

Table 3.8 *Personal Pronouns (Possessive)*

number	person		
	1st	**2nd**	**3rd**
singular	*mine*	*yours*	*his, hers, its*
plural	*ours*	*yours*	*theirs*

Consider the following utterance:

the book is *Graham's*

The proper noun *Graham* is said to be in the genitive case when it is displayed as *Graham's*. This simply means that it is signalling possession, ie, the book belongs to Graham. In the following utterance, the noun *dog* is also in the genitive case, ie, the bone belongs to, or is possessed by, the dog:

that is the *dog's* bone

Possessive pronouns, therefore, substitute for genitive nouns. The previous two examples can be reformulated as follows:

the book is *his*
that is *its* bone

Further examples of the use of possessive pronouns are shown below:

the book is *mine*
I think the choice is *hers*, don't you
theirs is a selfish way to act

Reflexive Pronouns

Reflexive pronouns refer to the same person, or thing, as the subject of an utterance. The complete set is shown in Table 3.9.

Table 3.9 *Reflexive Pronouns*

number		person	
	1st	2nd	3rd
singular	*myself*	*yourself*	*himself, herself, itself*
plural	*ourselves*	*yourselves*	*themselves*

Consider the following:

<u>he</u> only has *himself* to blame

In this utterance the subject is *he* and the reflexive pronoun that refers to the *he* is *himself*. In the following example, the subject is *they* and the reflexive pronoun that refers to *they* is *themselves*:

<u>they</u> must do it *themselves*

Here are a few more examples:

<u>the creature</u> gorged *itself*
<u>Martine</u> smiled to *herself*
<u>the players</u> gave *themselves* a lot of problems

Demonstrative Pronouns

Table 3.10 *Demonstrative Pronouns*

	proximate	non-proximate
singular	*this*	*that*
plural	*these*	*those*

Demonstrative pronouns include the same members as those identifiers that are demonstrative, ie, *this, that, these* and *those* (see Table 3.5). The difference in usage is that when these words are functioning as pronouns they are substituting for nouns. Consider the following utterance:

this is a book

In this instance, *this* is substituting for the noun *book*. Therefore, in this context *this* is a demonstrative pronoun. Now consider the following:

this book

In this utterance, *this* is serving to identify the book as one that is close by. There is no noun for which it is substituting. So it is functioning as an identifier. As with demonstrative identifiers, demonstrative pronouns serve to point out something, or some things, that are either proximate (*this*, *these*) or non-proximate (*that*, *those*). Further examples of demonstrative pronouns include:

this is a fast-moving train   [*the Inter City Express is a fast-moving train*]

that is a great movie   [*Sixth Sense is a great movie*]

I'll have to see about *those* [*I'll have to see about the pictures*]

Interrogative Pronouns

Pronouns such as *who, whom, whose, what,* and *which* that substitute for nouns in particular questions are referred to as interrogative pronouns (see Jackson, 1990). Consider the following question and answer sequence:

1   *who* is that?
2   that is Graham

From this sequence we can see that the *who* in the first utterance is substituting for the noun *Graham*, as evidenced in the answer of the second utterance. In this context, therefore, *who* is considered to be a pronoun, as it is substituting for a noun (*Graham*). Consider a further example:

1   *what* is she playing?
2   she is playing chess

Again we can see that the interrogative *what* in the first utterance is substituting for the noun *chess*, as provided in the answer of the second utterance. Once more, in this particular context, the word *what* is described as an interrogative pronoun because it is substituting for a noun (*chess*). Here are some further examples:

whose is this?	[*it is <u>Mary's</u>*]
which is yours?	[*the <u>box</u> is mine*]
you gave it to *whom*?	[*I gave it to <u>Bob</u>*]

Indefinite Pronouns
There is a final set of words that are referred to as pronouns, but they differ from all of the pronouns discussed so far in that they do not substitute specific nouns. This set includes the following: *no-one, anyone, someone, everyone, nobody, anybody, somebody, everybody, nothing, anything, something* and *everything*. Consider the following utterance:

he gave it to *no-one*

In this utterance the word *no-one* is used because the person referred to is unknown or indefinite. We cannot argue that this pronoun is substituting for a specific noun (eg, *he gave it to <u>Rupinder</u>*) because the person remains unknown. Consider a further example:

something brushed my leg

Again we see that the word *something* is used because it refers, in this instance, to some indefinite, non-personal animate or thing (see Jackson, 1990, 42). Once more, it cannot be argued that this word is substituting for a specific noun (eg, *the <u>ball</u> brushed my leg*), because the thing is unspecified, ie, it is indefinite. Further examples of indefinite pronoun usage include the following:

everyone knows that I am a good son-in-law
anything can happen in the next half hour
he gave her *nothing*

Prepositions
Prepositions function as relation words that connect elements of an utterance together. Consider the following:

the colour *of* money

In this utterance, the word *of* is the preposition. It connects one noun, *colour*, with another, *money*. However, the word *of* in this context does not have any individual meaning. It is only meaningful in the context of connecting the two nouns in the utterance. Other examples of prepositions connecting nouns in this way include the following:

	Noun	Preposition	Noun
a	book	*for*	Sanjeev
the	sound	*of*	music
a	churn	*for*	butter

As well as connecting to a noun, or pronoun, prepositions can also connect to a verb:

	Verb	Preposition	
Rutger	went	*to*	the festival
he	flew	*with*	his friends
Karen	worried	*about*	Nina

Finally, prepositions may also connect to an adjective:

	Adjective	Preposition	
Anil was	late	*for*	the meeting
her touch was	soft	*on*	his skin
Jeff was	cruel	*with*	her

Conjunctions

These words conjoin, or add together, one element with another. There are two types: coordinating, and subordinating.

Coordinating Conjunctions

Conjunctions such as *and*, *but* and *or* typically serve to add together two elements that are perceived to be of equal status. Consider the following utterance:

> bread *and* butter

Here, the two elements *bread* and *butter* may be perceived to be equal, one is not subordinate to the other. The conjunction that coordinates these two elements is *and*. Similarly, the two elements *my books* and *your cassettes* are also perceived to be on the same footing in the following utterance:

my books *or* your cassettes

This time the conjunction *or* is used to coordinate the two elements. In contrast to the use of *and*, which implies addition, the conjunction *or* typically implies selectivity, ie, one of the elements or the other, but not both. Further similar examples include the following:

knife *and* fork
not the knife *but* the fork
the man *or* the woman

Subordinating Conjunctions

In contrast with coordinating conjunctions, conjunctions such as *since, if, because, so, when, as* and *though* subordinate one element to another, ie, they imply some sort of condition or contrast. Consider the following:

I'll do it *if* you do it first

The second element of this utterance, *you do it first*, is subordinate to the first element, *I'll do it*, as the conjunction *if* signals a condition, ie, I will only carry out this action if, and only if, you carry out the action first. The following utterance provides a further example of a contrast between two elements:

I'm nervous *although* I think I can do it

The first element, *I'm nervous*, indicates the speaker's psychological state, ie, they are is nervous. This state is contrasted with the subordinate second element, *I think I can do it*, which expresses another psychological state, ie, the belief that he or she can carry out some particular action, despite the fact that he or she is nervous. Further examples of subordinating conjunctions include the following:

she can leave *when* she starts acting properly   [condition]
they all cried *since* they had all loved the dog   [contrast]
Graham will have to go now *because* the train is
about to leave   [condition]

This concludes our description of the nine word classes of English. For convenience, the foregoing outline is summarised in Figure 3.1.

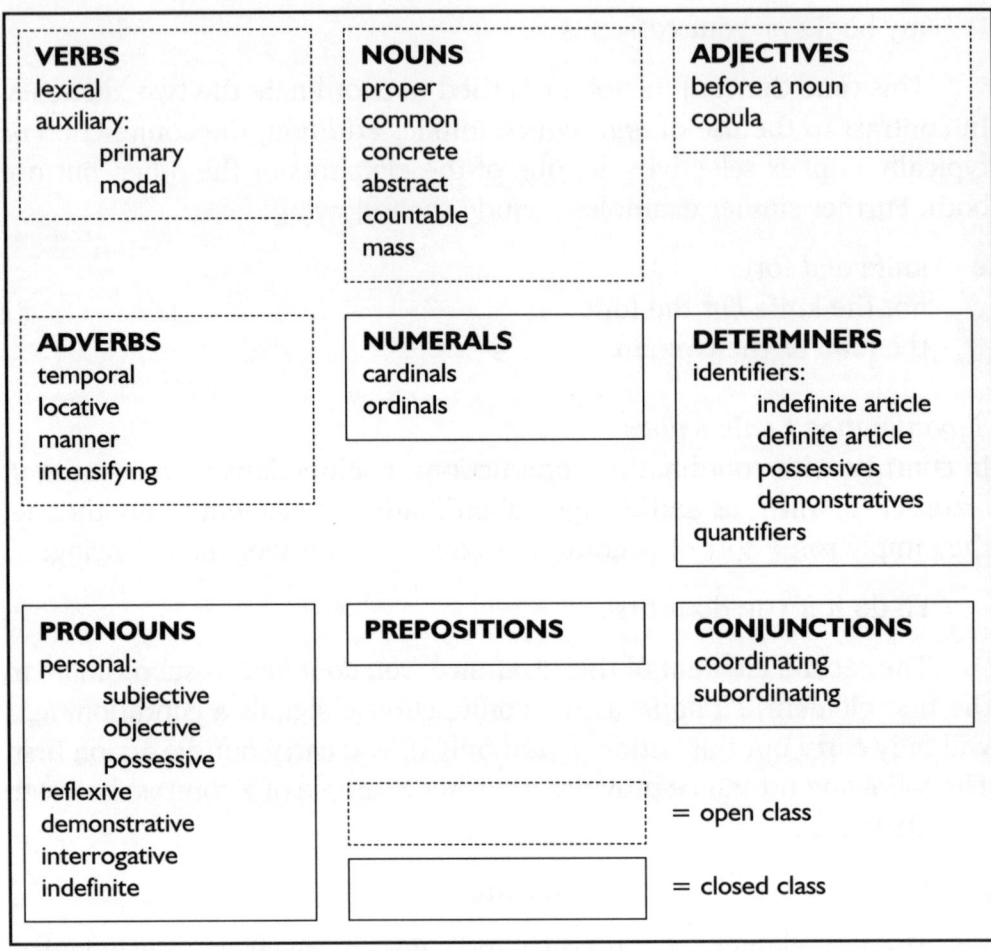

Figure 3.1 *The Nine Word Classes of English*

In this chapter we have considered the key language property of duality, that is, how units at the primary level of organisation are constructed from elements at the secondary level of organisation. What we have not yet fully explored is that each level has its own principles of organisation, rules that govern how elements and units can be combined and sequenced. This leads us to the notion of syntax and this is the subject of the next chapter.

Revision Exercises

3.1 What is the difference between an open and a closed word class?

3.2 Identify the bound (B) and free (F) morphemes in the following utterances – eg, *they*(F) *re-*(B)*negotiate*(F)*-ed*(B) *the*(F) *term*(F)*-s*(B):

> *his disinterest showed when I replayed the singing detective videos*
> *if you reconsider I will happily provide some inexpensive watches*
> *the priests determined that their lives were preordained*

3.3 Identify the word class (verb, noun, adj, adv, num, det, pron, prep, conj) to which each of the words in the following utterances belongs – eg, *the* (det) *boy* (noun) *hugged* (verb) *the* (det) *dog* (noun) *and* (conj) *the* (det) *cat* (noun):

> *she drank the red liquid quickly*
> *yesterday, Margaret gave it to him*
> *three men cried because they were very unhappy*
> *the furry cat jumped in the large yellow box*
> *the first girl and her friend left for home*
> *quietly, quietly, the little mouse crept*
> *the right man*
> *a man on the right*
> *may I be the first to congratulate you*

Activities

3.4 Audio-record a five-year-old child in conversation with an adult. Identify, as far as possible, all conjunctions used by the child. What type of conjunction (coordinating, subordinating) predominates? Can you suggest why?

3.5 Make a suitable length audio recording of (a) a three-year-old child talking to their peers, (b) an adult in conversation with another adult. Transcribe the first 200 words spoken by the selected child and the selected adult. Now analyse each word and identify the word class to which it belongs. Make a chart that shows the number of verbs, nouns, adjectives, adverbs, numerals, determiners, pronouns, prepositions and conjunctions used. Compare the results for the child with those for the adult. Are there any major differences in distribution? Can you explain any differences?

CHAPTER 4

Combining Words

IN THE PREVIOUS CHAPTER we explored the key language property of duality, ie, how elements at the secondary level of organisation combine to form units at the primary level of organisation. We noted how morphemes combine to form words. We also considered how words that all perform the same function group into classes. In this chapter we examine another key property of language – structure-dependence. We have already seen that structure-dependence implies that language possesses an underlying patterned structure. Specifically, the primary units of language, the words, appear to combine according to set rules. These rules are known as syntactic rules, and we begin our discussion in this chapter by defining syntax as the rules that govern the combination of words, and their sequential placement, in order to create meaningful utterances. Then we describe the manner in which words combine to compose larger units known as phrases. Five phrase types are discussed: verb phrase, noun phrase, adjective phrase, adverb phrase, and prepositional phrase. Next, we examine how these five phrases may be combined into yet larger units known as clauses. The seven clause structures of English are examined, and the issue of what constitutes a sentence, and what constitutes a well-formed clause is broached.

Sequencing Rules

We have noted that syntax concerns itself with the rules that govern which words may be related to form meaningful utterances, and in what order. To illustrate, what does the following word mean?

blind

The two most common interpretations of meaning would probably be either, 'without the power of sight' or 'a screen for a window'. Now, what does this word mean?

Venetian

Did you interpret this as meaning 'a native or inhabitant of Venice'? Perhaps you again considered it to mean, 'a screen for a window'? But now consider the following:

Venetian blind

Is this the same as the following?

blind Venetian

It should be obvious that a Venetian blind is not the same as a blind Venetian!

Venetian blind ≠ blind Venetian

This simple example illustrates very well the notion of syntax. It is apparent that the correct sequencing of words is crucial to convey the appropriate meaning. In the case of *Venetian blind* the noun *Venetian* serves to modify the noun *blind*, to create a new composite noun *Venetian blind*, a process known as noun modification. In the instance of *blind Venetian*, the word *blind* is seen to be functioning as an adjective that qualifies the noun *Venetian*. Syntax, then, is concerned with the inter-relationships of words. Another example is provided by the utterance *light night*, where it is also apparent that a *light night* is not the same as a *night light*, ie:

light night ≠ night light

In the case of *light night*, we see that *light* is functioning as an adjective that qualifies the noun *night*. In the utterance *night light*, the

95

noun *night* serves to modify the word *light*, which is here functioning as a noun. Therefore this is another example of noun modification to produce the composite noun *night light*. We see that a change to the sequential order of the words creates a change in the meaning of the utterance. A final example should consolidate the notion that syntactic rules define the appropriate sequencing of words in order to create particular meanings. Consider the following:

Danish cheese ≠ cheese Danish

The word *Danish* in the utterance *Danish cheese* is functioning as an adjective that qualifies the noun *cheese*. It is describing a particular type of cheese. However, in the utterance *cheese Danish*, the word *Danish* is functioning as a noun, ie, the name of a particular type of pastry confectionery. We see, once more, that the noun *cheese* in the utterance *cheese Danish* is functioning as a noun modifier, ie, it describes the type of pastry as being one that contains cheese.

It is apparent that words may belong to more than one word class. One of the determinants that defines which class a word belongs to is its sequential placement in an utterance. So, for example, we have seen that *blind* is an adjective in the utterance *blind Venetian*, but that it is functioning as a noun in the utterance *Venetian blind*. In all the examples provided so far, each of the sequences is acceptable, although they convey different meanings, ie:

Venetian blind
blind Venetain
light night
night light
Danish cheese
cheese Danish

However, while all of the above two-word sequences are acceptable, not all two-word sequences are acceptable. Consider the following brief exercise:

> Using only the word 'happy', see how many grammatically correct utterances you can make by adding just one more word
> (eg, happy *hour*)

What do you notice about all the words you have added to the word *happy*? If the utterance is to make sense, and is to appear complete, then the only words that can be added are those that are functioning as nouns, eg:

happy *mother*
happy *dog*
happy *birthday*

It is not possible in English to add adverbs to the word happy. For example:

happy *curiously*
happy *strangely*
happy *rather*

Similarly, it is not possible to add prepositions to it:

happy *out*
happy *between*
happy *through*

Further, it is not possible to add adjectives to it to form meaningful two-word utterances:

happy *blue*
happy *strange*
happy *wonderful*

In summary, except for the combination of <u>adjective + noun</u>, the above two-word combinations are not syntactically correct in English.

Syntactic rules, then, prescribe which words can be associated with which other words in a language, and in what order. In the case of a two-word utterance beginning with an adjective, the syntactic rule states that only a noun can be appended. Any other class of word is syntactically incorrect. While sequences such as <u>adjective + adverb</u>, <u>adjective + preposition</u>, and so on, are unacceptable as a two-word utterance spoken in isolation, this is not to say that such sequences can never exist in English. Consider, for example, that although the combination <u>adjective + adjective</u> is unacceptable in a two-word utterance, this same combination can exist in a meaningful way in certain four-word utterances, eg:

the <u>happy blue</u> bird
my <u>happy strange</u> friend
your <u>happy wonderful</u> wife

Similarly, while the sequence <u>adjective + preposition</u> is unacceptable in a two-word utterance spoken in isolation (eg, *happy on*, *happy about*, *happy for*), this sequence can appear in certain longer utterances, eg:

Jill is <u>happy on</u> the floor
I am <u>happy about</u> it
he was <u>happy for</u> you

So, syntactic rules apply not only to the immediate environment (whether or not two words can be combined together), but also to the context of occurrence, ie, while certain word combinations may not be allowable on their own, in longer utterances they may be acceptable in the context of other word combinations. In the later section that examines phrases, we will look at some of the rules that govern how certain groups of words may be combined to form acceptable constructions. Before this, however, we will make a brief comment on the sequencing of morphemes.

Sequencing Morphemes

So far in this section we have considered only how whole words may be sequenced in order to create meaning. We have seen how, if one does not follow the rules of syntax, then the resulting word combination may be rendered meaningless. In just the same way that sequencing rules apply to words, similar sequencing rules also apply at the morphological level.

Recall that in the previous chapter we considered how one might add prefixes and suffixes to the root morpheme *organise*. It is apparent that there is an accepted sequential order for the addition of bound morphemes to free morphemes. So, the following sequences are acceptable:

re-organise
dis-organise

However, the following constructions are not permitted by the sequential rules governing the placement of bound morphemes:

organise-re
organise-dis

In other words, *re-* and *dis-* may only function as prefixes, they may not be appended as suffixes. Similarly, the bound morphemes *-ed*, *-er*, *-ation*, *-ing* and *-s* may only function as suffixes, ie:

organis-ed
organis-er
organis-ation
organis-ing
organise-s

Any other sequential placement of these bound morphemes is not permitted by the syntactic rules that govern the placement of morphemes. Consequently, each of the following sequences is unacceptable in English:

ed-organise
er-organise
ation-organise
ing-organise
s-organise

Phrases

In this section we outline the ways in which words may be combined to form larger units known as phrases. Five phrase types are introduced: (1) verb phrase, (2) noun phrase, (3) adjective phrase, (4) adverb phrase, and (5) prepositional phrase. First, consider the following utterance:

the boy hugged the dog

Notice that the words in this syntactically correct structure combine into three units: (1) *the boy*, (2) *hugged*, and (3) *the dog*, ie:

the boy	hugged	the dog

These units remain unbroken even if the surface structure is rearranged, while at the same time retaining the same meaning, eg:

the dog	was hugged by	the boy

These units are known as phrases. Phrases represent an intermediate level of organisation between the word and what is known as a clause, ie, words do not combine immediately into clauses but, rather, into smaller units known as phrases. We introduced this concept in Chapter 2, where we considered the structure-dependence of language. We also noted that it is possible to change elements of phrases, eg:

the girl	hugged	the dog
the man	hugged	the dog
the soldier	hugged	the dog

the boy	*washed*	the dog
the boy	*kicked*	the dog
the boy	*worried*	the dog

the girl	hugged	the girl
the man	hugged	the man
the soldier	hugged	the soldier

In addition, the phrases can be modified and expanded, eg:

the big boy	had hugged	the cowering frightened dog
the ever-present boy	was hugging	the somewhat large dog
the rather naughty boy	may hug	the clean dog

It should be evident that these phrases could be expanded and amended almost indefinitely. However, we have also seen that there are limitations on which words may be combined with which others. We will now highlight some of the more important features of English phrases, through a consideration of the five major phrases in English usage, beginning with the verb phrase.

Verb Phrases

The simplest verb phrase (VP) consists of just a head verb, which is always a lexical verb. So, returning to our earlier example of *the boy hugged the dog*, the verb phrase is simply the head lexical verb *hugged*. This can be represented diagrammatically by using what is known as a tree diagram:

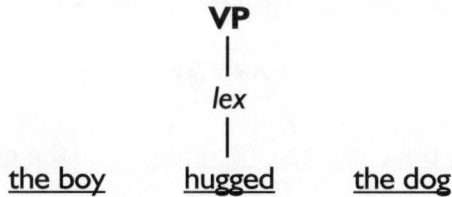

The head lexical verb in a verb phrase may, however, be modified by the addition of auxiliary verbs.

Pre-Modifying Auxiliaries

Recall that the main auxiliary verbs are *be* and *have*. Auxiliary verbs in verb phrases always precede the head lexical verb, ie, they are pre-modifiers. So, for example, our utterance may be modified through the use of the auxiliary *be*, as represented by the following tree diagram:

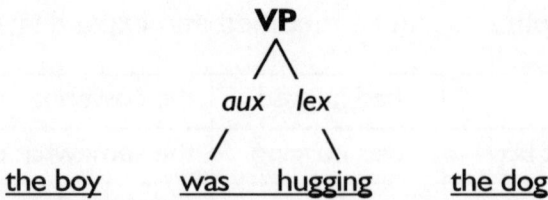

Similarly, it may be modified through the use of the auxiliary *have* as shown below:

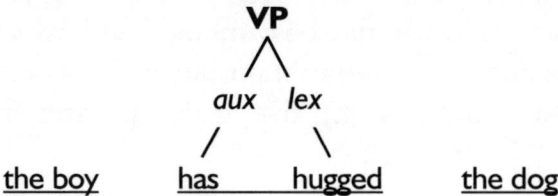

In addition to the primary auxiliary verbs *be* and *have*, recall that there is also a small set of modal auxiliaries. These indicate the mood or attitude of the speaker and include items such as *can, could, should, must* and *may*. Again, returning to our primary example, this could be modified as follows:

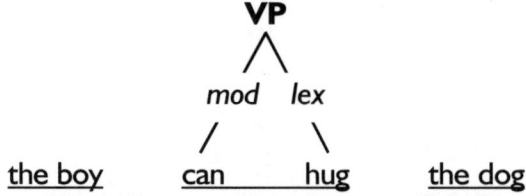

It is, of course, also possible that a head lexical verb may be modified by both a modal and primary auxiliary verb, for example:

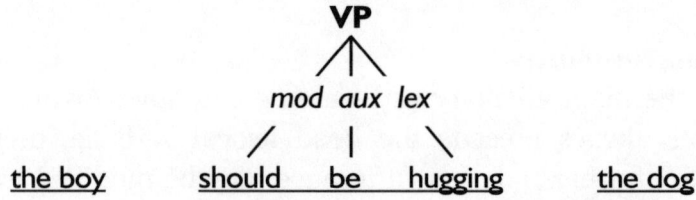

Noun Phrases

As with verb phrases, noun phrases (NP) must consist minimally of a head. This may be either a noun or a pronoun, for example:

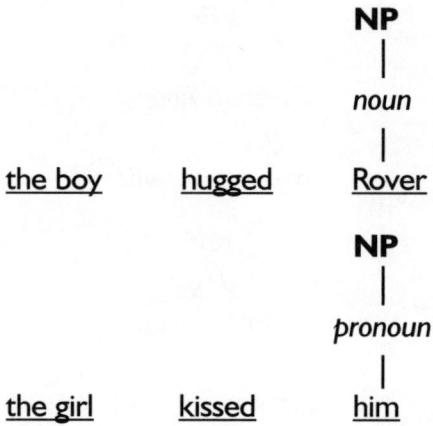

The head in noun phrases may also receive pre-modification. There are five main ways this may be achieved. It may be pre-modified by (1) identifiers, (2) numerals, (3) quantifiers, (4) adjectives, and (5) adjectives and their associated intensifying adverb. We will now provide examples of each of these types of modification, using our original utterance *the boy hugged the dog* as a baseline.

Pre-Modifying Identifiers

In our example utterance, *the boy hugged the dog*, there are actually two noun phrases, as indicated below:

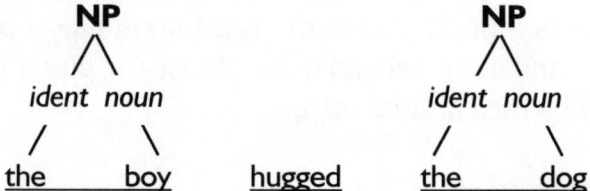

The head in each noun phrase is a noun (*boy, dog*), and in each case it is modified by the identifier *the*. This is, of course, the definite article. However, any of the identifiers (indefinite article, definite article, possessives and demonstratives) may be used to pre-modify the head noun. Here are a couple of examples. The first uses the possessive identifier *my* to pre-modify the head noun *wife*, and the second uses the demonstrative identifier *this* to pre-modify the head noun *book*:

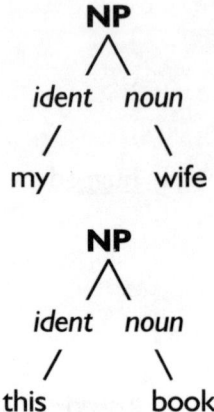

Pre-modifying numerals

Consider the following modifications to our baseline utterance:

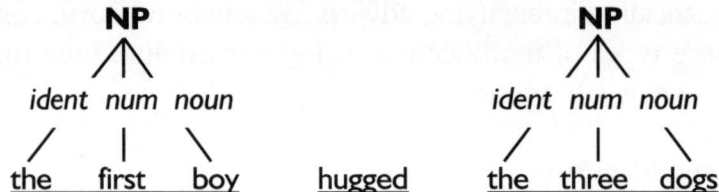

We see that the head nouns in each of the two noun phrases of our baseline utterance have now been pre-modified by the insertion of a numeral. In the first noun phrase the head noun *boy* is pre-modified by the ordinal *first*, and in the second noun phrase the plural head noun *dogs* is pre-modified by the cardinal *three*.

Pre-Modifying Quantifiers

Recall that quantifiers such as *several*, *few* and *many* are used to make reference to indefinite quantities. In the following example both head nouns in each of the noun phrases in our baseline utterance have been pre-modified by the use of a quantifier. The first is the quantifier *several* and the second is the quantifier *various*:

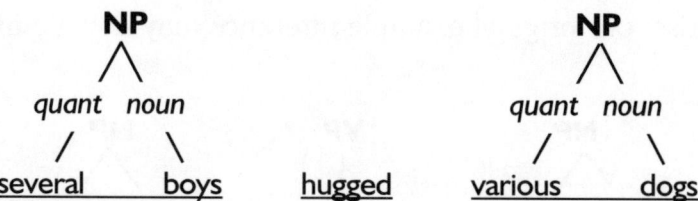

Pre-Modifying Adjectives

We saw in the previous chapter that adjectives are descriptors that qualify nouns by providing additional and specific information. We also noted that they commonly occur before a noun. The reason for this should now be apparent, ie, because they may be used to pre-modify a head noun, but not to post-modify the noun. In the following example, the head of the first noun phrase is pre-modified by the adjective *happy*, and the head of the second noun phrase is pre-modified by the adjective *sad*:

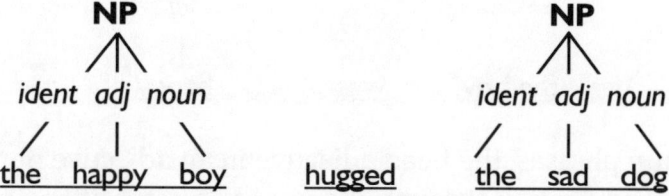

Pre-Modifying Adjectives and Associated Intensifying Adverb

In the previous chapter we saw how certain adjectives appear to be gradable and that they can, therefore, be modified by an intensifying adverb. For example, *quick* is a gradable adjective as it can be modified by intensifying adverbs to produce utterances such as *very quick*, *extremely quick*, *rather quick*, and so on. Similarly, *distraught* is a gradable adjective as it too can be modified by an intensifying adverb, eg, *greatly distraught*, *severely distraught*, *somewhat distraught*. So it is possible to pre-modify head nouns with both an adjective and its associated intensifying adverb, for example:

```
        NP                          NP
       /|\                         /|\
 ident int adj noun          ident int adj noun
  /  /  |  \                  /   |   \  \
the very happy boy   hugged  the rather sad  dog
```

To summarise, our original example utterance may now be illustrated as follows:

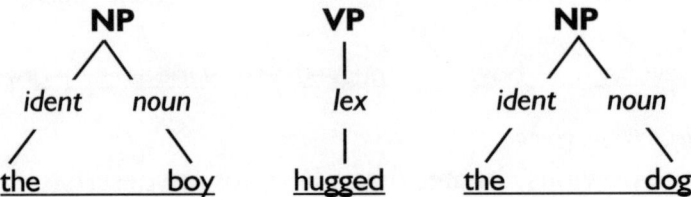

Adjective Phrases

As the name implies, adjective phrases (AdjP) have an adjective as the head, for example:

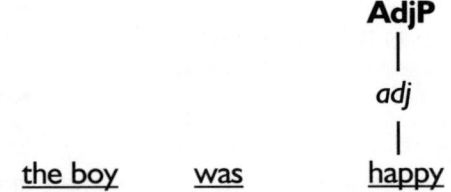

Like noun phrases, the head adjective in an adjective phrase can also receive pre-modification through the use of an intensifying adverb.

Pre-Modifying Intensifying Adverbs

We have already seen that intensifying adverbs are capable of modifying gradable adjectives. For example, *quiet* is a gradable adjective that can be modified by a preceding intensifying adverb, eg, *very quiet, rather quiet, moderately quiet*. The adjective *soft* is another example of a gradable adjective that can be modified by intensifying adverbs to produce utterances such as *very soft, fairly soft, reasonably soft,* and so on. We noted in the previous chapter that intensifying adverbs always precede their associated adjective, and the explanation for this should now be obvious, ie, it is because they function as pre-modifiers in adjective phrases. Here is an example of the use of the intensifying adverb *very* to pre-modify the head adjective *happy*:

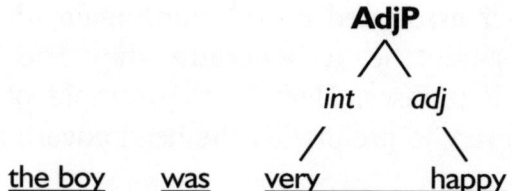

A further example should suffice to illustrate this usage:

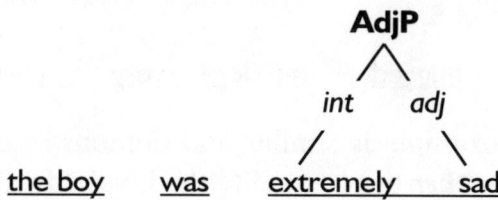

This is a fairly straightforward example in which the intensifying adverb *extremely* is used to pre-modify the head adjective *sad*.

Adverb Phrases

The head of an adverb phrase (AdvP) is, of course, an adverb, for example:

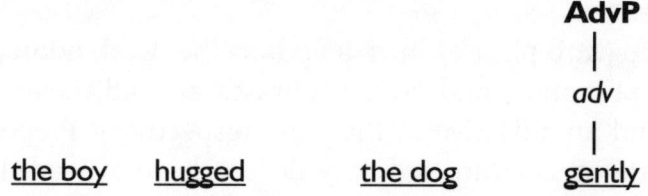

As with noun phrases and adjective phrases, the head of an adverb phrase can also be pre-modified by the use of an intensifying adverb.

Pre-Modifying Intensifying Adverbs

We have seen that intensifying adverbs are capable not only of modifying adjectives, but of modifying other gradable adverbs. For example, *quietly* is a gradable adverb that can be modified by a preceding intensifying adverb, eg, *very quietly, rather quietly, extremely quietly*. The adverb *softly* is another example of a gradable adverb that can be modified by intensifying adverbs to produce utterances such as *very softly, fairly softly, quite softly*, and so on. We noted in Chapter 3 that intensifying adverbs always precede their associated adverb and, again, the reason for this should now be apparent, ie, it is because they also function as pre-modifiers in adverb phrases. Here is an example of the use of the intensifying adverb *very* to pre-modify the head adverb *gently*:

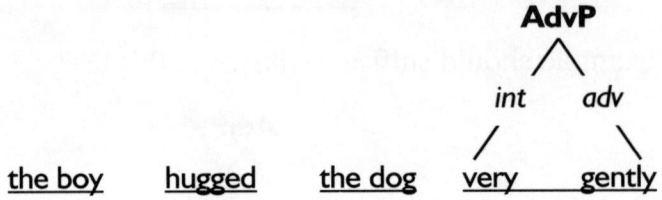

The following example is similar and demonstrates the use of the intensifying adverb *rather* to pre-modify the head adverb *tightly*:

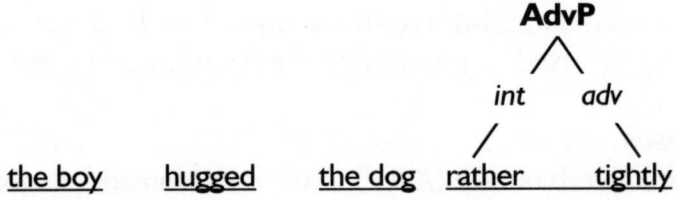

Prepositional Phrases

We have noted how verb phrases have a verb as the head, noun phrases have a noun (or pronoun), and adverb phrases and adjective phrases have an adverb and an adjective as the head respectively. Prepositional phrases (PrepP) are unusual in that they do not have a head. Instead, they have two compulsory elements, a preposition and a noun phrase. Consider the following:

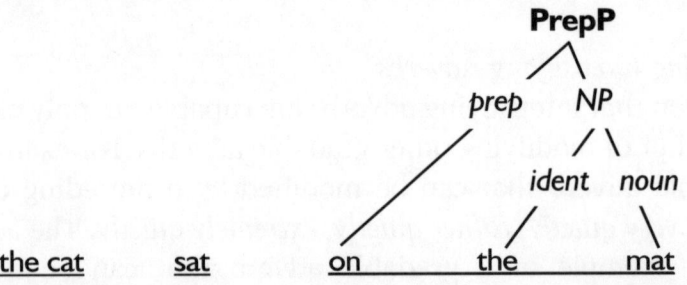

The prepositional phrase is only complete if both the preposition and noun phrase are combined. That is to say, neither *the cat sat on*, which omits the noun phrase, nor *the cat sat the mat,* which omits the preposition, would be correct. Consider a further example:

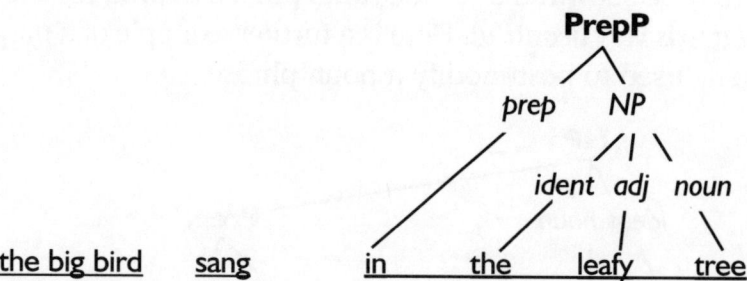

In this example we see that the two compulsory elements, a preposition and a noun phrase, are in evidence. Again, one without the other would make the utterance nonsensical, ie, neither *the big bird sang in,* omitting the noun phrase, nor *the big bird sang the leafy tree,* omitting the preposition, would be acceptable. Now, because prepositional phrases have no head they cannot be pre-modified. However, prepositional phrases themselves can be used as post-modifiers of noun phrases, ie, they may follow the head noun in such phrases.

Post-Modification of Noun Phrases
Consider the following example of a noun phrase in which a prepositional phrase is used to post-modify the head noun:

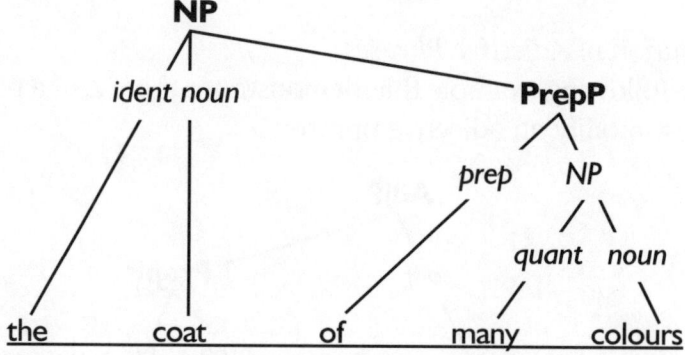

The noun phrase is *the coat of many colours* and the head noun is *coat.* This head noun is pre-modified by the identifier *the.* In addition, it is post-modified by the prepositional phrase *of many colours.* It is a simple matter to determine if this complex structure is functioning as a complete noun phrase, as it is always possible to substitute a pronoun for a whole noun phrase. So, in the utterance *the coat of many colours was beautiful* a pronoun may be substituted for the noun phrase to produce the modified utterance *it was very beautiful*. Here is a further example of a prepositional phrase being used to post-modify a noun phrase:

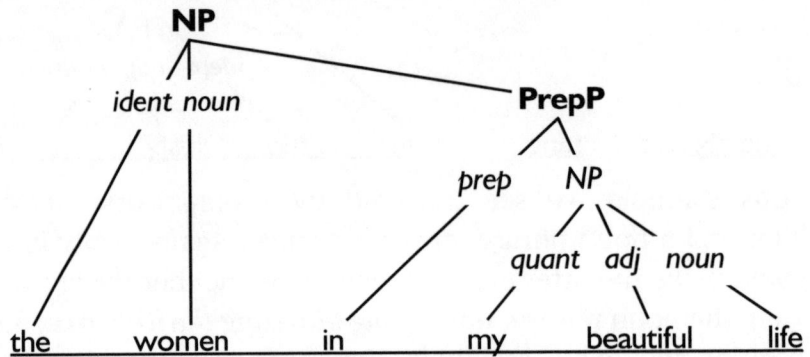

The noun phrase is *the women in my beautiful life*, the head noun being *women*. As before, it is pre-modified by the identifier *the* and post-modified by a prepositional phrase. The prepositional phrase *in my beautiful life* consists, as it should, of both a preposition (*in*) and a noun phrase (*my beautiful life*). Not only can prepositional phrases be used to post-modify noun phrases, however, they can also be used to post-modify adjective phrases.

Post-Modification of Adjective Phrases
Consider the following example that demonstrates the use of a prepositional phrase to post-modify an adjective phrase:

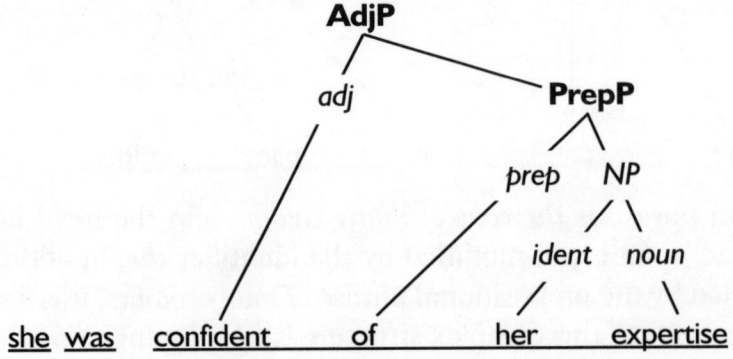

The adjective phrase is *confident of her expertise* and the head adjective is *confident*. It is this head adjective that is post-modified by the prepositional phrase *of her expertise*. This prepositional phrase consists of the compulsory preposition (*of*) and noun phrase (*her expertise*). A further example of post-modification of an adjective phrase with a prepositional phrase is shown below:

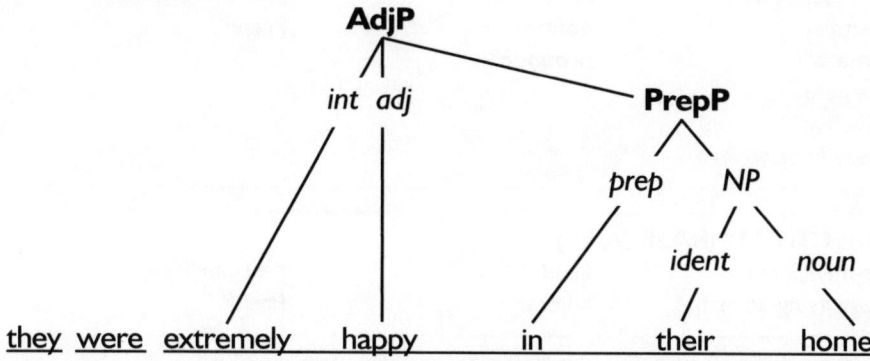

In this example, the adjective phrase is *extremely happy in their home*. The head adjective is *happy* and we see that this has been both pre- and post-modified. It is pre-modified by the intensifying adverb *extremely* and post-modified by the prepositional phrase *in their home*. This prepositional phrase, once more, consists of the two compulsory components of a preposition (*in*) and a noun phrase (*their home*). There are actually several other ways in which noun phrases and adjective phrases may be post-modified, but space does not permit a more detailed discussion. However, the examples provided should be sufficient to demonstrate how words are combined into the larger phrasal units of language. Figure 4.1 overleaf summarises the structure of all the phrases we have discussed in this section.

VERB PHRASE (VP)

pre-modification	*head*
auxiliary verb	lexical verb
modal auxiliary	

NOUN PHRASE (NP)

pre-modification	*head*	*post-modification*
identifier	noun	PrepP
numeral	pronoun	
quantifier		
adjective		
intensifying adverb		

ADJECTIVE PHRASE (AdjP)

pre-modification	*head*	*post-modification*
intensifying adverb	adjective	PrepP

ADVERB PHRASE (AdvP)

pre-modification	*head*
intensifying adverb	adverb

PREPOSITIONAL PHRASE (PrepP)

preposition + NP

Figure 4.1 *The Structure of English Phrases*

Clauses

We have seen how words combine into five types of phrase in English, ie, verb phrase, noun phrase, adjective phrase, adverb phrase and prepositional phrase. These phrases are then further combined to construct larger units known as clauses. Phrases function differently in different clauses and we begin this section by considering the various functions of phrases. We then outline the different types of clause structure that arise from various combinations of phrases. Finally, we consider what constitutes a sentence and discuss the concept of a well-formed clause.

The Function of Phrases

Phrases function in different ways when combining to create clauses. There are five functions: (1) Subject, (2) Verb, (3) Object, (4) Adjunct, and (5) Complement. Each of these functions will be defined briefly below.

Subject

The Subject (S) is the thing or person performing the action, and it is noun phrases that typically function as Subjects in clauses. So, in our example of *the boy hugged the dog* the Subject is *the boy*, ie, it is the boy who is performing the action of hugging. Similarly, in the utterance *Rebecca was drinking the milk*, the Subject is *Rebecca*, as it is she who is performing the action of drinking. We see, therefore, that in both examples the Subject was represented by a noun phrase, ie, *the dog, Rebecca*.

Verb

The Verb (V) describes actions that are instigated by someone or some animate being, events that happen, or the state people or things are in. The verb function is invariably represented by a verb phrase. So, in *the boy hugged the dog*, the Verb is represented by the verb phrase *hugged*, which consists of just the lexical verb that describes the action performed by the boy. Similarly, in the utterance *Rebecca was drinking the milk*, the Verb function is represented by the verb phrase *was drinking*, which consists of a pre-modifying auxiliary verb *was* and the head lexical verb *drinking*.

Object

The Object (O) is the thing undergoing the action and this function is, like the Subject, typically represented by a noun phrase. So, in *the boy hugged the dog*, the Object is *the dog*, ie, it is the dog that undergoes the action of hugging. Similarly, in the utterance *Rebecca was drinking the milk*, the Object function is represented by the noun phrase *the milk*, as it is the milk that has undergone the action of being drunk.

Adjunct

The Adjunct (A) provides additional circumstantial information about the time, location, manner, or cause of an action, event or state. This function is commonly represented by adverb phrases, although noun phrases and prepositional phrases may also function as Adjuncts. Adjuncts are usually optional elements, as their removal does not normally interfere with the meaning of the clause. There is no Adjunct in the clause *the boy hugged the dog*. However, if we were to say *the boy hugged the dog yesterday* then the adverb phrase, consisting of the head adverb *yesterday*, functions as an Adjunct. In this instance, it provides additional information related to time, ie, it specifies when the action of hugging the dog took place. Similarly, in the utterance *Rebecca was drinking the milk very quickly*, the Adjunct function is represented by the adverb phrase *very quickly*, which consists of the intensifying adverb *very* and the head adverb *quickly*. This Adjunct also provides circumstantial information about the manner in which Rebecca drank the milk.

Complement
A complement (C) fills the same position as an Object in a clause, and this function is usually represented by an adjective phrase or a noun phrase. It will be easier to understand the difference between an Object and a Complement after we have considered some of the clause structures of English. We will return to an explanation of this function later, in the section on SVC structure.

Clause Structure
Seven basic clause structures are identifiable in English: (1) SVO, (2) SV, (3) SVA, (4) SVC, (5) SVOC, (6) SVOA, and (7) SVOO. Each of these will be discussed in turn below.

SVO Structure
English syntax generally follows a Subject-Verb-Object (SVO) order. Consider once more the following example.

the boy hugged the dog

We have already commented that the Subject of the clause (the thing or person performing the action) is *the boy*; the Verb, which describes the particular action, is *hugged*, and the Object (the thing undergoing the action) is *the dog*. Therefore this clause can be represented as follows:

Subject	Verb	Object
the boy	hugged	the dog

We have also noted how both the Subject and Object are represented by noun phrases, and that the Verb is represented, as it must always be, by a verb phrase. Further examples of the basic SVO structure include the following:

Subject	Verb	Object
my dad	washed	his car
your friend	was opening	the door
Verity	is throwing	a ball

The basic SVO structure of English syntax can be modified in a number of ways, but there are two main methods. The first is to remove or replace a functional element, and the second is to add another functional element to the three-part structure. The SVO structure and its variants are known as clauses. We will now consider a further six ways in which the basic SVO structure of English is modified.

SV Structure

The basic Subject-Verb-Object structure can be reduced to produce a clause with the structure Subject-Verb (SV), for example:

Subject	Verb
Anila	kicked
my mother	is drilling
the girl	laughed
Li Wei	went

A point to note here is that some verbs may take an Object, and thereby be expanded into the basic SVO structure, whereas some may not. Consider the first example *Anila kicked*. This SV structure could be expanded into an SVO structure as follows:

Subject	Verb	Object
Anila	kicked	the ball

Similarly, the second example *my mother is drilling* could also be expanded into an SVO clause, for example:

Subject	Verb	Object
my mother	is drilling	a hole

Verbs such as *kick* and *drill* that are capable of taking an Object are referred to as transitive verbs. However, not all verbs are capable of taking an Object. Consider the verb *laugh* in the third example *the girl laughed*. It is not possible to expand this utterance into an SVO structure, for example:

Subject	Verb	
the girl	laughed	it

It is evident that this utterance is syntactically incorrect because *laugh* is incapable of taking an Object. Similarly, the verb *go* in the fourth example *Li Wei went* is also not capable of taking an Object. So, for example, the following construction is also syntactically incorrect:

Subject	Verb	
Li Wei	went	it

Verbs such as *laugh* and *go* that do not take an Object are known as *intransitive verbs*.

SVA Structure

The Object in the basic SVO structure can be substituted by an Adjunct that supplies further detail about actions, events and states. Adjuncts are most often optional elements that provide information related to manner, time, location or cause. Consider the following:

Subject	Verb	Adjunct	
the small child	cried	very loudly	[Adjunct of manner]
my friend	left	that evening	[Adjunct of time]
Sarah	lives	in America	[Adjunct of location]
she	has been sad	since you left	[Adjunct of cause]

We noted earlier that Adjuncts may be represented by adverb phrases, noun phrases and prepositional phrases. From the above examples, the Adjunct of manner in *the small child cried very loudly* is represented by the adverb phrase *very loudly*. Further examples of Adjuncts represented by adverb phrases include the following:

Subject	Verb	Adjunct (AdvP)
Beckham	played	superbly
my charming son	was hovering	rather sheepishly
she	would behave	so bravely

From the previous examples, the Adjunct of time in *my friend left that evening* is represented not by an adverb phrase but by a noun phrase, *that evening*. Further examples of Adjuncts represented by noun phrases include the following:

Subject	Verb	Adjunct (NP)
the boy	ran	two miles
your fourth cousin	sang	this afternoon
Ravi	shouted	that morning

The Adjunct of location in *Sarah lives in America* from the earlier examples is represented by a prepositional phrase, *in America*. Further examples of prepositional phrases functioning as Adjuncts include the following:

Subject	Verb	Adjunct (PrepP)
Robert	ran	to the door
Helen's brother	played	after his dinner
the ball	was bouncing	on the pitch

SVC Structure

We noted earlier that a Complement may fill the same position as an Object in a clause. However, there is a fundamental difference between an Object and a Complement when the Complement replaces the Object in a SVO clause. The difference is that the Subject and Object refer to different things, whereas the Subject and Complement (in a SVC clause) refer to the same thing. Consider the following:

Subject	Verb	Object
Julie	stroked	the cat

In this clause, the Subject refers to one thing (*Julie*) and the Object refers to another thing (*the cat*), ie, they are not the same. In contrast, the Subject and Complement refer to the same thing, for example:

Subject	Verb	Complement
Dawn	seems	happy

In this clause, the Complement (*happy*) makes reference to the same thing as the Subject (*Dawn*), ie, it is Dawn that is happy. Other examples include the following:

Subject	Verb	Complement (AdjP)
Brian	went	mad
this book	is	terrible
my mother	appeared	sad

It should be apparent from all of these examples that the Complement refers to the same thing as the Subject, ie, Brian is mad, the book is terrible, the mother is sad. In all the examples provided above, the Complement has been represented by an adjective phrase consisting of just a head adjective (*mad, terrible, sad*). However, we have indicated that Complements may also be represented by noun phrases. For example:

Subject	Verb	Complement (NP)
the witch	changed into	an ant
Adam	was born	a hero
Kathryn	became	the dentist

Again we see that the Subject and Complement refer to the same thing, ie, the witch is the ant, Adam is the hero, Kathryn is the dentist. In each of these examples, the Complement is represented by a noun phrase made up of an identifier and a head noun (*an ant, a hero, the dentist*).

SVOC Structure
Recall that, as well as removing or replacing an element in the basic SVO structure, we can also add other elements. One possibility is to append a Complement, ie, SVOC. We have seen that when a Complement fills the same position as the Object in the SVO structure then the Complement

refers to the same thing as the Subject. However, the Complement refers to the same thing as the Object when it follows the Object. For example:

Subject	Verb	Object	Complement
Paul	considered	your ideas	very silly

It is apparent in this example that the Complement (*very silly*) refers to the same thing as the Object (*your ideas*), ie, it is the ideas that are very silly and not Paul that is very silly. Other examples include the following:

Subject	Verb	Object	Complement
Cole	found	the game	frustrating
the mussels	made	Rupinder	ill
Daniel	imagined	Anna	much taller

In each of these examples we see that the Object and the Complement refer to the same thing, ie, it is the game that is frustrating and not Cole that is frustrating; it is Rupinder who is ill and not the mussels, and it is Anna who is imagined to be much taller and not Daniel.

SVOA Structure

As well as adding a Complement to the fundamental SVO structure, we can also add an Adjunct. Recall that Adjuncts are discretionary elements that supply extra information related to manner, time, location, and so on. Consider the following:

Subject	Verb	Object	Adjunct
the boy	hugged	the dog	gently

In this utterance the Adjunct function is represented by an adverb phrase that consists of just the head adverb *gently*. This Adjunct provides gratuitous information regarding the manner in which the Subject, *the boy*, carried out an action on the Object, *the dog*. We now realise that this action was carried out gently. Here is a further example:

Subject	Verb	Object	Adjunct
the man	held	the woman	so gently

In this clause, the Adjunct is again represented by an adverb phrase, this time consisting of the head adverb *gently* which is pre-modified by the intensifying adverb *so*. Once more, this is an Adjunct of manner that describes how the Subject, *the man*, performed the action of holding on the Object, *the woman*. Here are some further examples of SVOA structures:

Subject	Verb	Object	Adjunct	
Megan	wrote	her essay	quickly	[Adjunct of manner]
the therapists	assessed	the children	yesterday	[Adjunct of time]
Daniel	cleaned	his flat	in London	[Adjunct of location]

SVOO Structure

The final English clause structure involves the addition of a second Object to the primary SVO structure, ie, SVOO. When two Objects are included in a clause a distinction is made between the direct object (O_d) and the indirect object (O_i). The direct object is the thing or person undergoing an action, being talked about, etc, and the indirect object is the person who is the recipient or beneficiary of the action. Consider the following example:

Subject	Verb	Indirect Object	Direct Object
Nadia	gave	her mother	a beautiful card

In this example, the thing undergoing the action is *a beautiful card*, ie, it is the card that is being given. Therefore this is the direct object. The person who benefits from the action is *her mother*, ie, the beautiful card is given to the mother. Therefore this is the indirect object. Consider a further example:

Subject	Verb	Indirect Object	Direct Object
Graham	sent	Margaret	his love

In this clause the thing undergoing the action of being sent is *his love*, ie, it is Graham's love that is being sent. Therefore this is the direct object. The recipient of the action is *Margaret*, ie, she is the one who receives Graham's love. Therefore this is the indirect object. Further examples of SVOO clauses are given below:

Subject	Verb	Indirect Object	Direct Object
Alex	sent	Ryan	his regards
the twins	shipped	their friends	the carved clock
Sheila	tossed	Amerjit	my shuttlecock

To summarise, there are seven major clause structures in English. These are shown in Table 4.1.

Table 4.1 *The Clause Structure of English*

clause structure		example
Subject Verb	SV	*the bride* *smiled*
Subject Verb Object	SVO	*the bride* *kissed* *her husband*
Subject Verb Adjunct	SVA	*the bride* *smiled* *happily*
Subject Verb Complement	SVC	*the bride* *seemed* *happy*
Subject Verb Object Complement	SVOC	*the wedding* *made* *the bride* *happy*
Subject Verb Object Adjunct	SVOA	*the bride* *kissed* *her husband* *tenderly*
Subject Verb Object Object	SVOO	*the bride* *gave* *her husband* *a kiss*

These structures represent the major clause types in English. Nevertheless, because language is so flexible, we find variations of these clauses. For example, it is possible to have OSV structures such as the following:

Object	Subject	Verb	
Margaret	I	kiss	(but Susan I do not)
the dogs	David	likes	(but the cats he does not)
a cup	she	prefers	(but a mug she does not)

However, these sorts of constructions are often perceived to be a stylistically contrived variation of the basic SVO structure. The most pervasive variation, however, is the construction of clauses that incorporate adjuncts. Because adjuncts provide circumstantial information they can be appended almost indefinitely. Consider the following:

	Subject	Verb	Object			
	John	drew	the picture			
	Subject	**Verb**	**Object**	**Adjunct**		
	John	drew	the picture	carefully		
Adjunct	**Subject**	**Verb**	**Object**	**Adjunct**		
yesterday,	John	drew	the picture	carefully		
Adjunct	**Subject**	**Verb**	**Object**	**Adjunct**	**Adjunct**	
yesterday,	John	drew	the picture	carefully	with Kathy	
Adjunct	**Subject**	**Verb**	**Object**	**Adjunct**	**Adjunct**	**Adjunct**
yesterday,	John	drew	the picture	carefully	with Kathy	in the afternoon

This simple example demonstrates how adjuncts can be added to the basic SVO structure to create longer and longer clauses. All of the above, except for the first SVO structure, would be considered variations of the SVOA structure.

What is a Sentence?

We have seen that each higher order unit of organisation in language is constituted from elements of the immediately lower unit of organisation. We see that morphemes combine into words, that words combine into phrases and that phrases combine into clauses. What then is a sentence? Intuitively we might argue that a sentence is a unit of organisation larger than a clause. For most purposes this somewhat crude definition will suffice. In written texts, for example, it is fairly easy to identify sentences: they begin with a capital letter and end with a full stop! Even so, there is no universal agreement as to how long or short a sentence may be. Writers, and editors of texts, tend to divide sentences into manageable sizes, usually influenced by the amount of information that they consider the reader will be able to retain while reading the sentence. In other words, the sentence is divided into 'semantic chunks', units of meaning that appear to convey a complete thought. Therefore there are no commonly accepted rules that govern the structure of a written sentence.

A similar argument may also be applied to spoken language. We can be definite about the seven clause structures of English and note that all English clauses possess a verb. SO we may conclude that the possession of a verb is a defining characteristic of a clause. In addition, we can identify ways in which various clauses may be combined with others. For example, the use of the conjunction *and* is a relatively simple way of creating spoken utterances larger than a single clause:

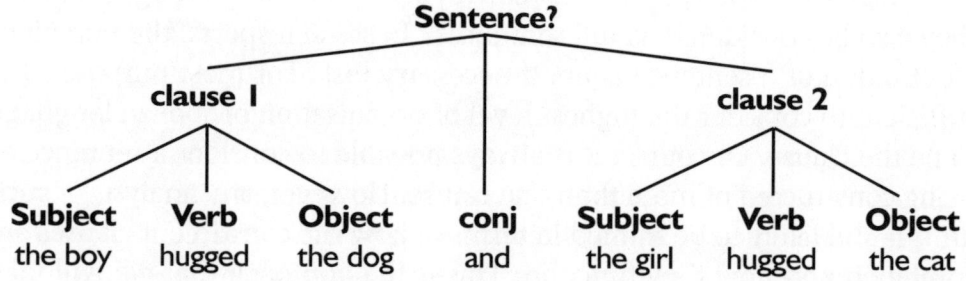

Rather like written texts, however, there are no rules that prescribe how long a spoken sentence may be. One would suppose that similar cognitive constraints would apply, ie, the listener would be able to retain and process only so much information in the auditory memory. With respect to the example provided above, it would be possible to link a whole string of SVO clauses through the coordinated use of *and*: eg, *the boy hugged the dog <u>and</u> the girl hugged the cat <u>and</u> the man ate the apple <u>and</u> the woman ate the orange* … and so on. There are no structural rules that limit the size of a so-called sentence. Nevertheless, even with this rather contrived example, it is possible to see some sort of semantic division. The clauses *the boy hugged the dog* and *the girl hugged the cat* appear to express a thought on the same theme and may be thought of as one sentence. Similarly, the two clauses *the man ate the apple* and *the woman ate the orange* also appear to express a unity of thought. The important point to note here is that it is not possible to define a spoken sentence by appealing to the form of an utterance. Our attempts at definition appear to be slightly more fruitful, however, when we appeal to the concept of meaning, ie, when we make a judgement about how the series of words conveys a speaker's complete thought. In addition, as we have noted, speakers typically vary the length of their utterances. For example, they may be heard to shout *stop!* Should this be considered a full sentence, as it conveys a complete thought? As well as using single words, speakers may also utter phrases: eg, in response to the question *who is this?* a speaker might respond *my dad*. This noun phrase similarly conveys the meaning of a complete thought, but should it be considered as a full sentence? There are also many examples of speakers producing single clauses, eg, *he gave it to me, that is mine, she came today*. Each of these clauses is interpretable as conveying a complete thought. Should they also be considered as full sentences? In some respects, the pursuit of a definition of a sentence is not a necessary task. For most purposes it is sufficient to consider the highest level of organisation of spoken language to be the clause. Of course, it is always possible to consider a sentence as being constructed of more than one clause. However, any analysis of such units is still likely to be framed in terms of how the constituent clauses are combined and how they function. This is the approach that we will take in this book, ie, that it is unnecessary to invoke the notion of a sentence in order to describe human language. Moreover, we will use the term 'utterance' to describe any meaningful vocalisation or vocalisations. As we have seen, a meaningful utterance could consist of merely a single word, a phrase, a clause, or a combination of clauses.

The concept of 'well-formed' clauses

You may have noticed that when we have been discussing certain phrases and clauses we have used terms like 'grammatically correct', 'syntactically correct' and 'unacceptable'. These terms have been used to describe the notion of a phrase or clause as being either 'well-formed' or 'not well-formed' with respect to the grammatical rules of English. In other words, does the construction of the phrase or clause conform to the rules of English grammar? If it does, it is considered to be 'well-formed'. If it does not then it is considered to be 'not well-formed'. It is argued that native speakers of English are able to make intuitive judgements about how well-formed a phrase or clause is. Indeed, in order to validate some of our discussions of correct and incorrect constructions we have appealed to your own intuitions as a means of endorsing our arguments. There is a danger, however, of assuming that because an utterance is well formed then it must necessarily be meaningful. Consider the following famous example proffered by the linguist Noam Chomsky:

colourless green ideas sleep furiously

This utterance is syntactically well-formed. In fact, it conforms to the syntactic rules of English regarding the formation of SVA clauses, ie:

Subject	Verb	Adjunct
colourless green ideas	sleep	furiously

However, it is meaningless. The following clause, derived from the above example, as well as being meaningless is also now not well-formed:

furiously sleep ideas colourless green

A second point to note is that our concept of 'well-formed' is influenced by the fact that we live within a literate society. In other words, we tend to consider an utterance as being well-formed in relation to how we would expect it to appear in a written text. But consider the following:

did they not deal in scandal surely

This construction was uttered by a radio presenter in conversation with a studio guest. As a written text it appears somewhat cumbersome and possibly ungrammatical. However, within the context of a relatively informal face-to-face conversation it is fairly typical of the sorts of incomplete and 'ungrammatical' constructions people make. Consider the following extract from a conversation between two adult males:

John: I think we're going for a full fortnight
Tony: for a full fortnight ... yeah
John: yeah
Tony: cos it's usually only a week, isn't it?
John: yeah
Tony: cos it's usually quite good, isn't it?
John: cos ... er ... last year ... er ... went to Salou and lost one of the lads up there ... and ... er ... we come back ... and one of the lads who I don't know about ...
Tony: oh, that's right ... yeah ... I remember, yeah ... I remember hearing about that
John: yeah
Tony: yeah ... bit unfortunate that
John: yeah ... so ...
Tony: yeah

Notice that this extract is full of hesitations, pauses and utterances that, according to the prescriptions of English syntax, would be considered 'not well-formed'. However, this extract is typical of much of our day-to-day use of language. We must recognise, therefore, that there is a difference between the sort of grammar that may be taught in schools, and to foreigners learning the language, and the grammar of actual native speakers in informal settings. These are known as prescriptive grammars and functional grammars respectively. So far, throughout the book we have been outlining the prescriptive grammar of English. Some aspects of a functional grammar will be discussed in the next chapter when we consider pragmatics, or the social use of language. As we begin the next chapter we will turn our attention to the meaning of linguistic tokens such as words, phrases and clauses under the rubric of semantics.

Revision Exercises

4.1 Define syntax.

4.2 Construct tree diagrams to represent the following underlined phrases, identifying the type of phrase (VP, NP, AdjP, AdvP, PrepP) and the word class and/or subcategory of the words that comprise them, eg, *the yellow custard*:

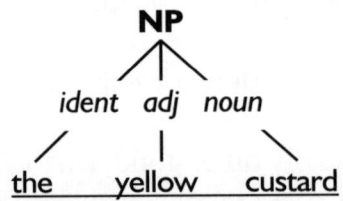

my happy mother
the girl *was kissing* her mother
the light was *extremely bright*
it fell *on the floor*
her friend *ran*
several books
she rode *in my new car*

4.3 Analyse the following clauses, indicating the function and type of phrases that comprise them, eg, *the boy* (S:NP) *kicked* (V:VP) *the ball* (O:NP) *quickly* (A:AdvP):

his sister called his mother
Lucy played happily
Margaret gave Graham a Valentine card
the dog barked
your mother sent a letter
Adele was reluctant
the two therapists taught the child in Darlington
the song made Kathryn happy

Activities

4.4 Look up definitions of *sentence* and *clause* in at least five different dictionaries. Then attempt to construct your own definition of a sentence.

4.5 Make a suitable length recording of an adult speaking (eg, from a news report on the radio or television) and transcribe at least 100 utterances. Identify, as far as possible, all the adjuncts used in each utterance. Construct a chart showing the function of each adjunct (time, location, manner, cause), and indicate the number of times each function occurs. Note which type of phrase (AdvP, NP, PrepP) is used to represent each Adjunct function. Finally, determine whether or not the speaker demonstrates a preference for placing Adjuncts at the beginning or the ends of their utterances.

5

Language Meaning & Language Use

THIS CHAPTER BEGINS WITH AN OVERVIEW of semantics – the study of the meaning of linguistic tokens. Some of the key principles are examined through a consideration of the part that semantic development plays in a child's development of early language skills. First, the notion of the holophrase is introduced, ie, single words used by infants to mean many different things. Second, we consider how misunderstanding may arise owing to the natural processes of over- and under-extension. Third, we introduce the concept of semantic categories, and demonstrate how children up to the age of 3;00 years relate semantic categories in their efforts to create longer, more specific utterances. We then turn our attention to pragmatics, the social use of language. We begin this discussion by considering the ways in which people can shift their style of communication to suit the social occasion. The various means by which syntax, morphology, vocabulary and phonology may be varied from the prescriptive rules of English are then outlined. Subsequently, we consider how certain aspects of our social interactions may be conscious or unconscious, and how particular variations are time-limited. The chapter concludes with a discussion of the dominance of male reference in the English language, a concept known as genderlect (Griffin, 1996).

Catch the Moggie!

Carry out the following brief exercise:

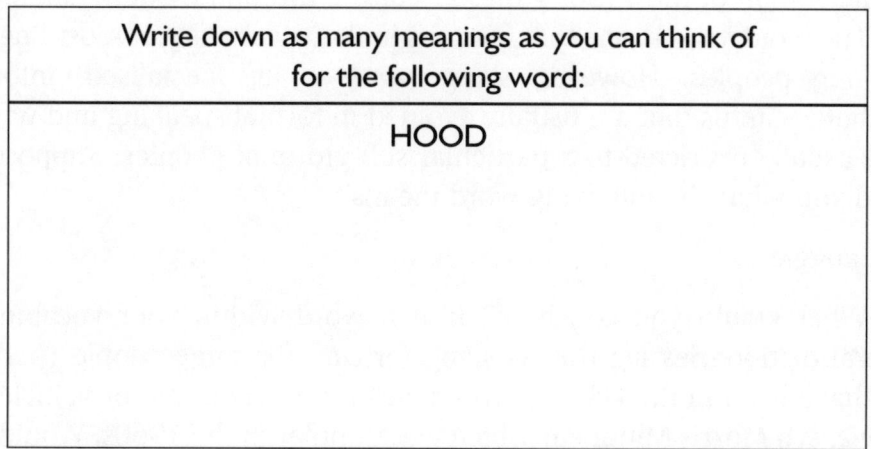

Write down as many meanings as you can think of for the following word:
HOOD

How did you do? Just what does *hood* mean? Well, your answer(s) to this will depend on a number of factors. Your interpretation will be influenced by such things as your age, your gender, where you live, your profession, your academic background, and so on. Some possible interpretations are:

1 a covering for the head and neck
2 the folding, waterproof canopy of a baby's pram
3 the hinged metal cover over the engine of a car
4 a lawless member of a gang of criminals

For English-speaking British people interpretation 1 is probably the most apparent. The term used to refer to a head covering has a long history, but it is still a term that is used today – even with respect to modern sports wear. Interpretation 2 is, perhaps, slightly less obvious. Modern, lightweight prams are somewhat different from the heavier, more robust, designs of the 1960s, and they do not always have a traditional folding hood. Perhaps the term is less well used nowadays to refer to parts of prams? Interpretation 3 is most readily associated with American English. British speakers tend to use the term *bonnet* to refer to the lid of a car engine. Clearly, for British speakers of English another interpretation of *bonnet* would also be 'a covering for the head'.

Interpretation 4 is again an American English term, and one that is largely not in use today. However, it is a well-known interpretation owing to the popularisation of the 1930s gangster culture through modern cinema.

The word *hood* is one that features in the vocabulary of most English-speaking peoples. However, slang words – ie, specialised, informal vocabulary items that are usually avoided in formal speaking and writing – are usually restricted to a particular sub-group of peoples. Suppose we asked you what the following word means?

moggie

What would you conclude? Is it a word within your vocabulary? Several dictionaries list this as slang for *cat*. For some people (perhaps who have lived in the UK and who have an interest in motor vehicles), a *moggie,* is a Morris Minor car which was popular in the 1960s. Would you have known this? How old are you? Where did you grow up? Did you own a Morris Minor? Again, who you are will influence your interpretation of words and whether or not the particular word is within your vocabulary. Finally, we have also been informed of a person in the Wirral, England who considered a *moggie,* to be a mouse. This anecdotal account illustrates very well the often idiosyncratic meanings assigned to certain words. Even though it might be generally accepted that *moggie,* is slang for *cat*, there may still be people who consider that it is not. The difference becomes an important one if this person is ordered to, 'Catch the moggie!'. Do they chase after the cat? The mouse? Or risk being run over by a car?

What is Semantics?

Semantics is the study of the meaning of linguistic tokens such as words, phrases and clauses (Gregory, 1999). It studies which signs are used, how they make reference to things, ideas, emotions, etc, and how the hearer interprets them. It considers such things as implication. For example, why is that if we say, 'Are you going to close the door?' this is interpretable as implying that the speaker is asking you to close the door and that they are not specifically enquiring as to whether or not you intend to close the door? In this situation a preferred response is that the listener either complies and closes the door, indicates their acknowledgement verbally before closing the door (eg, 'Oh, right'), or offers a token apology before closing the door (eg, 'Sorry'). Similarly, if we say to a toddler as a visitor is leaving, 'Are you going to wave bye-bye?', we usually do so to imply that the child should indeed wave bye-bye. It is not that we are specifically enquiring as to the child's intention. However, you are probably familiar with the situation where the toddler responds, 'No!'. In this situation the child appears to have made a literal interpretation. Similar confusions may arise over the use of proverbs and idioms, ie, generally accepted phrases that have a meaning different from the literal. An example is, 'Well, you might as well make hay while the sun shines.' Clearly, this phrase is not intended to mean that the listener should go and find a field of grass to mow in the summer sun. People with learning disabilities and some people who have suffered a stroke may have a great deal of difficulty interpreting proverbs and idioms. They tend to interpret many things literally. The field of semantics is complicated but, in order to demonstrate some of the principles, we will now consider the part that semantic development plays in a child's development of early language skills. This should provide an insight into what this field has to offer to our understanding of human communication.

The Holophrase

Recall that it is at the One Word Stage that we can appropriately talk about a child's expressive language. Recall also that at the Later One Word Stage (1;02–2;00 years) children begin to use a range of single words to refer to things in their environment or to actions, ie, they have a referential meaning. Now consider the following interaction between a child and its father:

child:	mummy
father:	that's right, mummy's coming home soon
child:	mummy!
father:	Er … you want to play with mummy?
child:	[pointing at hat] mummy
father:	Oh, you want mummy's hat?
	[child smiles as its father passes the hat]

Sequences like these are not uncommon, the young child repeatedly using just one word and the adult taking the burden of the conversation through a series of guesses until the correct response is made. Problems arise because, as adults, we tend to have fairly specific meanings for each of the words we use. For most adults *mummy* will probably refer to a female person. So if I say, 'Mummy' you will most likely think that I am referring to this person. However, as we have seen, things are not quite as straightforward as this when interpreting the utterances made by young children up to the age of about 2;00 years. In the above sequence, *mummy* had more to do with possession of an object than the name of a person, ie, the child pointed to a hat that belonged to mummy and uttered 'Mummy.' Thus, in this instance, the word *mummy* is not referring directly to the person but, rather, to an object that mummy possesses – the hat. We would, therefore, describe this child's utterance as having the function of possession. It is possible, of course, that the child could use the word *mummy* to refer to a person. Had the child intended this in the above sequence then the father's first response, *that's right, mummy's coming home soon* may have been correct. In this instance the word *mummy* would have had the function of naming.

Single words used by infants to mean many different things are called holophrases (Dore, 1975). For, although the child is producing only one word at a time, the words often have a composite meaning. We have noted, for example, that the word *mummy* could be used for naming a person or for indicating possession of an object. The confusion for the adult listener in interpreting holophrases arises, in part, because of the disparity between surface structure and deep structure (see Chapter 2). The child says *mummy* (surface structure), but the adult's understanding of the deep structure of this utterance is largely dependent upon the context in which it is spoken. In our example, the child's father only understood what was meant when the child eventually pointed to the hat, ie, the child supported its utterance through the use of non-verbal communication. Some indication of the various meanings of holophrases may, therefore, come from the child's facial expression, gesture, actions, and so on. In summary, holophrase refers to the fact that a single word is being used by the child to express a whole phrase that would normally be made up of several adult words. Let us now consider a few more examples (see Halliday, 1975).

Instrumental Function

The child may use a single word like *more* to indicate, 'I want some more cheese' or 'I want you to play with me some more'. Words that express the meaning, 'I want ...' or 'I need ...' are considered to function instrumentally.

Regulatory Function

A word such as *car* may have a regulatory function if its intended meaning is, 'Let's play with the car'. Words are considered to have this function if they are interpretable as the child indicating to the adult, 'Do as I tell you', ie, they regulate an adult's behaviour. So, the word *book* will also have a regulatory function if the intended meaning is, 'Let's read a book'.

Imaginative Function

This function is represented by words that can be interpreted by the adult as meaning, 'Let's pretend'. So, for example, if the child says, *woof!*, this may be intended to mean, 'Let's pretend that we are dogs'.

There are, of course, many more functions than the ones we have described here, but these few examples give a flavour of the various meanings that a single word can express. It also helps to explain why adults often misinterpret the talk of children up to the age of about 2;00 years.

Over- and Under-Extension

Another possible reason for adults' misinterpreting infants' talk is that some children use the same word to refer to many different objects. For example, the word *dog* may be used to mean all animals, whether or not the animal being referred to is a cat, a horse, a pig, or whatever. This is known as over-extension and it is very common during the One Word Stage. In the same way that some children use a particular word to refer to many objects or people, others restrict their use of a word that could appropriately be applied to many objects, people, etc, to only one or two things. For example, a child may use the word *drink* to refer solely to orange squash and not use the word at all to refer to milk, tea, lemonade, and so on. This is known as under-extension and this is also a common feature of the One Word Stage.

Beyond the Holophrase

The elegance of language development is that it is so logical. If I can express a meaning with just one word then, surely, I can express more with two? If I say *mummy* this may be ambiguous. But if I say *mummy gone* then the meaning is more specific. It is this extension beyond the One Word Stage that we will discuss in this section. Recall that at the later One Word Stage (about 1;02–2;00 years) the child is beginning to name objects in the environment. However, this ability is quite precarious at this stage. The ability to attach a label to an object may depend heavily on situational clues. For example, a child may be able to name its own cup which is blue and made of plastic and happens to be sitting on the child's high-chair table. However, the same child may, for example, be unable to name a yellow, china cup on the table in someone else's house. The point here is that the child may require consistent situational and contextual clues such as the location of an object, its colour, its size, what it is made of, and so on, in order to name it. If any of these clues are altered or removed the child may have difficulty in finding the right word to label the object. Eventually, however, at around 1;08–2;00 years of age, the child consolidates its use of single words, and two-word combinations begin to emerge. This is the Two Word Stage and it usually lasts until about 2;04–2;06 years.

Two Words Together

Anyone who has paid even the slightest attention to a young child's speech should be able to recognise two-word utterances similar to the following:

daddy car
mummy gone
find hat
more milk
where Katie
light off
shoe on
pretty coat

We noted in the previous chapter that many of these two-word combinations incorporate concrete nouns, eg, <u>mummy</u> gone, find <u>hat</u>, more <u>milk</u>, as these represent the important items in the child's environment. We also recognised that the child begins to combine words from different word classes, eg, *shoe on* = noun + preposition, *pretty coat* = adjective + noun. While it is true that the use of a two-word combination is a development beyond the use of just one word, nevertheless, the utterances may remain ambiguous. Consider, for example, the child who says *daddy car*. How should this be interpreted? Should we assume that the child is using it to signify possession, ie, 'this is daddy's car'? Or should it be understood as meaning 'daddy is in the car'? As with one-word utterances, two-word combinations are also heavily reliant upon the context for their interpretation. Once more, the adult will gather clues as to the child's intended meaning through the child's use of non-verbal components such as gesture, facial expression, etc, and the situation in which the utterance is made.

Semantic Categories

So far, we have examined two-word utterances by considering the types of word classes that may be combined, eg, noun + noun, noun + preposition, noun + verb, and so on. However, another method is to consider the various meanings that the words express, ie, to approach the problem semantically. The linguist Roger Brown (1973) has recognised several categories of meaning that all children seem to express. He called these categories semantic categories, which literally means 'meaning categories'. We will consider four of these: (1) agent, (2) object, (3) action, and (4) location.

Agent

Brown noted that children usually make a distinction between animate beings and inanimate objects. Animate beings are things that are alive such as dogs, cats, horses, people, and so on. All of these are capable of acting under their own volition. Brown used the term *agent* to describe the semantic category that includes words that refer to animate beings. Examples of *agent* words would include *mummy, daddy, Rover*.

Object

In contrast to animate beings, inanimate objects are not alive, and they are not capable of acting independently or of making decisions. The semantic category used to include all inanimate objects is simply labelled *object*. This category would include such things as *table*, *spoon*, *cup*, and so on.

Action
A third semantic category is that of *action*. Words in this category which express the idea of action include such words as *kick*, *run*, *bark*, and so on.

Location
Words in this semantic category express the notion of place. They may indicate where an *agent* or *object* is, or moves to, and where an *action* is performed. Examples include *garden*, *house*, *bath*.

Relating Semantic Categories
The two-word utterances that children produce are not the product of random combinations of words. Rather, children are systematic and logical in the way they combine words to express meaning. Roger Brown noted that children produce utterances by relating one semantic category to another. We will consider some of these next.

Agent + Action
A common relation found in the majority of children between the ages of about 1;08–2;06 years is that of *agent + action*. Consider the following:

agent	action
daddy	go

Here the word *daddy* represents an animate being, one that can act by its own will and make independent decisions. The word *go* expresses the meaning of an *action*, in this case 'going'. A further example is set out below:

agent	action
dog	bark

Again, *dog* refers to an animate being. While a dog may not be considered capable of making decisions in the same way as a human, it nevertheless is alive and can act independently. Therefore it is considered to be an *agent*. The word *bark* is another expression of an *action* – in this case, an action typically associated with a dog and not a daddy! Further examples include the following:

agent	action
mummy	run
bird	sing
horse	jump

Action + Object

Another common semantic relation is that of *action + object*. Consider the following example:

action	object
kick	ball

Here, *kick* is an *action* in the same way that *bark* was considered an *action* in *dog bark* and *go* was considered an *action* in *daddy go*. The inanimate *object* in this two-word utterance is clearly the *ball*. As mentioned earlier, the exact meaning that the child intends when uttering something like *kick ball* will still have to be gleaned from the context in which it is said. If the child is kicking the ball then this utterance may be intended to mean, 'I'm kicking the ball'. However, if the ball is on the floor in front of you and the child points to you and says, 'Kick ball!' then this may be meant as, 'You kick the ball now'. The first interpretation is more like the child describing what it is doing, and the second more like giving an instruction. Further examples of *action + object* include the following:

action	object
drink	milk
cut	paper
eat	dinner

Beyond Two Words

For most children the Two Word Stage is completed by 2;06 years of age. We have noted how logical and systematic child-language development is, so it should come as no surprise to learn that the next stage of development is that the child now adds a third word to the two-word combinations. This is the Three Word Stage. The two-word combinations are used as the building blocks for the longer three-word utterances.

(Agent + Action) + Location

Consider the earlier example of an *agent + action, daddy go*. Using this as the foundation, the child can expand it by adding a third semantic category. For example, the child may add the category of *location* as follows:

agent	action	location
daddy	go	home

Here, *home* represents a *location* to which daddy may go. The child has, therefore, expanded the *agent + action* combination to the longer and more specific *agent + action + location*. It is easy to see, then, how two-word combinations can be used as building blocks to produce a variety of different meanings by the addition of different *location* words. Further examples include:

agent	action	location
daddy	go	bed
daddy	go	work
daddy	go	school

(Action + Object) + Location

A similar development can be seen by reconsidering our earlier example of *kick ball*, which was described as an *action + object*. Again, the child can expand this two-word utterance by the addition of a *location* word. For example, the child could indicate where it wishes to kick the ball:

action	object	location
kick	ball	garden

Once again, *garden* represents a *location* word and the utterance has expanded from the two-word building block of *action + object* to *action + object + location*. Further examples include:

action	object	location
kick	ball	house
kick	ball	park
kick	ball	path

Obviously there are more possible combinations and expansions of two-word utterances than we have space here to consider. However, the examples provided should give some idea of the systematic and logical way in which children develop longer and longer utterances. An additional, and rather useful way, is by combining one or more utterances with the word *and*. We will consider this in the next section.

Lengthening the Utterance – the Use of 'And'

Consider the following brief encounter between Kate and a child:

Kate: What did you do on holiday?

child: We saw donkeys and we ate ice-cream and we played on sand and we…

Perhaps Kate regretted asking the question? The child's answer is a seemingly interminable chain of events. An answer to test anyone's patience. However, this example illustrates admirably how *and* is used to connect one utterance with another. Indeed, the use of *and* as a connector is one of the most pervasive ways in which children extend their utterances beyond the Two and Three Word Stages. The use of this short word is not as simple as it might first appear to be, however. Children use it creatively for a variety of reasons and we will consider four of these functions: (1) additive, (2) temporal, (3) causal, and (4) adversative (see Bloom, 1993).

Additive Function (2;01–2;03 years)

Consider again the child's response in the previous example:

We saw donkeys *and* we ate ice-cream *and* we played on sand *and* we …

You will note that each utterance which precedes an *and* is meaningful by itself. For example, *we saw donkeys* is understandable even if it is uttered on its own. Likewise, this is true of *we ate ice-cream*, and the utterance *we played on sand*. In other words, the combination created by chaining the utterances together with *and* does not produce a meaning that is anything other than the meaning of each independent utterance. This use of *and* to add independent utterances is referred to as the additive function. This usage may be construed as meaning the same as *also*, ie:

> We saw donkeys *also* we ate ice-cream *also* we played on sand *also* we …

It is generally accepted that children develop this use of *and* at around 2;01–2;03 years of age. Recall, however, that there is wide variation among children when developing linguistic skills. This is true of the acquisition of *and*, with some children using it earlier than 2;01 years and others not using it until considerably later than 2;03 years. However, one constant appears to be that, regardless of the age at which the word is acquired, children almost invariably use it first in its additive function. Further examples of this include the following:

> I write *and* I paint
> she is strong *and* she is tall
> mummy is nice *and* mummy is happy

This function is sometimes also referred to as 'pure' addition (see Quirk & Greenbaum, 1973, 257). However, it is not the only function that *and* assumes. From 2;02 to 2;08 years of age children begin to introduce concepts of time into their utterances, and to use *and* in its temporal function.

Temporal Function (2;02–2;08 years)

There are a number of ways in which children can express time. One of the most obvious is to use temporal markers such as *after, Monday, today, now* and so on. For example:

> I swim *after* dinner
> we go on *Monday*
> daddy is home *today*
> you play *now*

Alongside this use of temporal markers, children also begin to use *and* to mark such things as sequential events. Consider the following utterance:

I went to the shop *and* I came back

It may be assumed that *and* is displaying just the additive function here. After all, *I went to the shop* and *I came back* are both capable of standing alone as meaningful utterances. However, the combination utterance is more than an example of addition because its two constituent utterances are, in some way, dependent upon each other. The action of the second utterance, 'coming back', is dependent on the first action, 'going to the shop'. Thus, there is a sequential order to the combination utterance. First the child goes to the shop and then it comes back. It is self-evident that the child does not first come back and then go to the shop. In this context, we can see that *and* is used to mark a temporal function that is similar in meaning to *subsequently*, ie:

I went to the shop *subsequently* I came back

Other examples of the temporal use of *and* include:

I got up *and* I got washed
daddy read a book *and* he fell asleep
the horse fell *and* Kathryn cried

Each of these further examples could be described as additive. However, they also include an element of temporal continuity, ie, the second action follows on from the first. It is the fact that temporal utterances are usually also additive that explains why children use *and* in its additive function before they use it in its temporal function. If the temporal utterance involves both an understanding of addition and temporal sequence then it is, clearly, more complex than an utterance that requires only an understanding of addition. The last example above, *the horse fell and Kathryn cried*, is interesting because, as well as marking a sequential order to the events – ie, Kathryn cried after the horse fell – there is a sense in which it was the horse falling which caused Kathryn to cry. Consequently, as well as marking a temporal function, the use of *and* in this utterance also marks a causal function. Children begin to use this function at almost the same time they begin using *and* in its temporal function, ie, 2;03–2;08 years.

Causal Function (2;03–2;08 years)

As already mentioned, *and* can be used to signal that one event caused another event to happen. Its use demonstrates the child's growing awareness that certain events, or actions, have consequences. Consider the following:

> mummy kissed Ryan's knee *and* it felt better

This utterance demonstrates the child's awareness that one action, 'mummy kissing Ryan's knee', was the cause of a new state, 'the knee felt better'. The use of *and* in this context can often be interpreted as meaning *therefore* or *so*, ie:

> mummy kissed Ryan's knee *therefore* it felt better
> mummy kissed Ryan's knee *so* it felt better

Further examples include:

> mummy go home *and* Ruth is sad
> Adam kick the ball *and* the window break
> the bee stung *and* it hurt me

Look again at all the examples of the causal function. As well as *and* displaying the additive function – ie, connecting the two constituent utterances – it also displays the temporal function. In other words, all of the events of the second utterances happen after the events of the first utterances have taken place, ie, Ryan's knee feels better after his mummy has kissed it, Ruth is sad after her mummy went home, the window broke after Adam kicked the ball, and the child becomes hurt after the bee stings it. So, we see that the causal function also incorporates both the additive and temporal functions. Again, this explains why children develop the causal function after the temporal function, which in turn is developed after the additive function. There is a cumulative effect to the development of the use of these functions, each function being dependent upon the function that precedes it.

Adversative Function (2;05–2;11 years)

The fourth important use of *and* is to signal some sort of contrast between the first utterance part and the second. Consider the following example:

Robert is happy *and* Helen is sad

This utterance contrasts one state, 'Robert being happy', against another state, 'Helen being sad'. This use of *and* may be construed as meaning *but*, ie:

Robert is happy *but* Helen is sad

You may have expected from the discussion of the cumulative effect that all examples of the adversative function would include the additive, temporal and causal functions. Well, this is evidently not the case. In the example of *Robert is happy and Helen is sad*, the combination utterance only relies on adding the two utterance parts. There is no obvious sense in which Helen being sad can be thought of as necessarily following on in time from Robert being happy. Also, it is not apparent how Robert being happy would cause Helen to be sad. In summary, the use of *and* in this example demonstrates the additive and adversative functions, but not the temporal or causal functions. There are, however, examples of the adversative function displaying both the additive and temporal functions, for example:

I was sick *and* now I'm not sick

Clearly, this combination utterance adds together the two utterance parts, but it also displays an understanding that not being sick follows on from being sick, ie, it displays the temporal function. The combination also contrasts one state (being sick) with another (not being sick) and it is, therefore, another example of the adversative function. In summary, *and* here demonstrates the additive, temporal and adversative functions, but not the causal function. As you may have anticipated, we can also find examples of the adversative function which rely on an understanding of all of the preceding functions. Consider the following combination utterance:

the dog chewed the clean carpet *and* now the carpet is dirty

This complex utterance embraces all four functions. First, the two utterance parts are added, ie, *the dog chewed the clean carpet* is added to *now the carpet is dirty*. Second, the temporal function is demonstrated by the fact that the carpet being dirty follows on in time from the carpet being clean. Third, the causal function is demonstrated by the child's understanding that it was the dog chewing the carpet that caused it to become dirty. Finally, there is the contrast of the state of a clean carpet with that of a dirty carpet, which demonstrates the child's use of the adversative function. So, we see in this utterance how the one small word *and* can be used to signal a whole wealth of meaning.

What is Pragmatics?

Pragmatics is the study of the use of language in context (Verschueren, 1998). Recall that in our earlier discussion of grammar we noted a difference between a prescriptive grammar – ie, a set of rules that describes how speakers should produce 'proper', well-formed utterances – and a functional grammar – ie, a description of how native speakers actually use the language in everyday contexts. Prescriptive grammars are those which are commonly taught to pupils at school and to foreigners wishing to learn the particular language. In addition, prescriptive grammars are often advocated by people who take the view that language is in some way becoming corrupted, or that children are developing 'sloppy' English. A prescriptive grammar is characteristically viewed as the most appropriate and 'correct' definition of how English should be spoken and written. Functional grammarians, however, tend to be less interested in prescribing what is, and what is not, considered correct according to social mores than in describing how language is actually used.

Style-Shifting

Consider the following two utterances:

1   hoy us a stottie
2   would you pass the sandwiches?

The two utterances are quite distinct in terms of their grammar and vocabulary. The first is spoken in the Geordie, dialect of north-east England, while the second conforms more closely to the prescriptive English language. For those of you who are unfamiliar with Geordie, the meaning of the first utterance can be gleaned from reading the second utterance. This is because the two are essentially equivalent in meaning (*hoy* = to throw or to pass; *stottie*, = a type of soft, white bread). Moreover, the same person spoke both utterances. Which one do you suppose was uttered in an informal setting and which one in a formal setting? Most people tend to think that the first utterance is more informal than the second, rather formal request. In fact, the first utterance was overheard being spoken by a male teenager at a school party with his classmates, and the second by the same teenager at an inter-school buffet lunch with pupils and teachers from different schools whom he had never met before. It is a fairly common feature that the more standardised, prescriptive language tends to be spoken in formal settings. Most people exhibit this ability to shift the style of their communications to suit the occasion. The more prescriptive, standardised English is sometimes referred to as *acrolect* (higher language) and the more informal as *basilect* (lower language). These terms are somewhat confusing, however, as they may imply that basilect is not as creative or flexible as acrolect. This would be a mistake as basilect demonstrates immense variety and creativity with respect to syntax, morphology, vocabulary, and so on. Style-shifting is based on a speaker's assumptions regarding what is, and what is not, appropriate for a particular situation. Many things will influence these assumptions. Take a moment now to list some of the things you think might influence the way we choose to speak to others, ie, to adopt a formal or informal style.

factors influencing choice of style

There are many factors that influence our choice of style, and some of the factors that sway one person may not be a significant influence for another. For example, how often have you heard something like, 'I don't care if he is the boss, I treat everyone the same!'? This speaker appears to be declaring that occupational status is not a significant factor in influencing their choice of style. Having highlighted variability in the importance of different factors, some possible factors that might influence our choice of style include the following:

- the interactants' gender (male or female?)
- their perceived status (an important official? a child?)
- the topic of discussion (corporate business meeting? gossiping in the street?)
- the location (noisy swimming pool? doctor's surgery?)
- the perceived language ability of the listener (a toddler? a foreigner?)
- whether the topic is embarrassing or intimate (personal physical relationships? intimate medical details?)
- the relative ages of the interactants (adult-adult? adult-teenager? elderly person-child?)
- the medium of communication (spoken? written? telephone answering machine?)

This list is by no means exhaustive. Also, it is important to note that we are not usually influenced by just one factor at a time. Typically, a number of factors interact to influence our choice. A 37-year-old male speech and language therapist speaking to a female teenager about her articulation difficulties in a hospital clinic may choose quite a different style from a 37-year-old female accountant talking to her teenage son about her imminent separation from his father.

Varying the Prescription

The common, everyday use of language may be varied in several ways from the prescriptive grammar. The main alterations occur in relation to (1) morphology, (2) syntax, and (3) vocabulary. Clearly these three variations are related to language. While we have not yet fully begun our discussion of speech, it is worth noting a fourth variation at this juncture, related not to language but to speech. This is (4) phonology. Each of these will be discussed in turn.

Morphology

One fairly obvious example of morphological variation
distinction. Where *whom* would once have been considered co..
is now a tendency to use *who*. Consider the following variations:

for *whom* the bells toll
for *who* the bells toll

I shall give it to *whomsoever* I wish
I shall give it to *whoever* I wish

There is often variation in the use of *shall/will*, although English prescription is less clear about which is 'correct'. For example:

I *shall* have to leave soon
I *will* have to leave soon

Another similar example includes the *amongst/among* distinction:

from *amongst* the forest peoples
from *among* the forest peoples

Syntax

Consider the following:

I've took it
she's gave it to me

In these utterances the irregular simple past (*took* and *gave*) has replaced the irregular past participle (*taken* and *given*). According to English prescription this would be considered incorrect and the utterances should have been rendered as *I've taken it* and *she's given it to me*. However, this sort of variation is quite common in the Tees Valley area of the north-east of England.

Vocabulary

Vocabulary changes are the most common variation. They can be divided into four types: (1) slang, (2) jargon, (3) cant, and (4) interjections. Each of these will be considered in turn.

Slang

Slang consists of highly informal, non-standard words and phrases. These are often colourful expressions formed by the creative and playful organisation of words. Slang is generally avoided in formal speaking and writing. It usually has its origins within a particular subculture. However, if the subculture is in frequent contact with the mainstream culture then the slang words or phrases may become incorporated into the mainstream culture. Examples of slang words are *bog, john, loo* and *can* for 'toilet', *spondoolee, moola, bread* and *wad* for 'money' and *wheels* for 'car' (see Ayto, 1999; James, 1999).

Jargon

This is specialised vocabulary used by people in the same work or profession. The specialised words are ordinarily only partially understood by outsiders. Jargon is useful for people within particular professions because it allows members of that profession to communicate clearly and concisely with a minimum of ambiguity (see Burke & Porter, 1995). Examples of jargon within the speech and language therapy profession include *dyspraxia* (a vocal tract motor sequencing disorder of speech), *aphasia* (a complete inability to use language symbols in order to communicate) and *metathesis* (the interchange of segments in words, eg, when *tiger* becomes *giter*)

Cant

This is sometimes referred to as *argot* and it is the secret vocabulary of underworld groups. Examples of cant as used by gangsters include *snuff*, *blow away* and *waste* which mean 'to kill'. It should be apparent that the dividing line between slang, jargon and cant is quite tenuous. Words that begin as cant, such as *waste* and *snuff*, may eventually become slang as they are promoted throughout the mainstream culture through the cinema, novels, and so on.

Interjections

Interjections, or vocatives, are exclamations such as *oh, mm, uh huh, yeah* and *well*. They are frequently inserted into a conversation by the current listener to indicate attention and to acknowledge what is being said. In addition, they may be used to express an emotional reaction to what has been said, eg, *Really?* and *Well, I never!* They do not, therefore, function as grammatical elements in an utterance. There is some evidence to suggest that women are more prolific users of interjections than men, and that men and women use different types of interjections (Coates, 1993; Williamson, 1995). Moreover, there is a great deal of individual variation in their use, with some people favouring the use of just one or two types of interjection at the expense of others. Consider the following extract from a conversation between two males, T and J:

T: I've been various places in Spain … for two weeks
J: mm
T: and … er … erm … you know it's okay
J: yeah
T: the food's reasonable … the things are … a little …
J: mm
T: bit … a tiny bit more expensive … like they cost a few pesetas and that
J: yeah
T: it's like a hundred and seventy-five pesetas to the pound
J: yeah
T: but I mean … I'm sure Yvette can handle that
J: yeah
T: the things that are luxuries like …
J: yeah
T: Kit Kats and things …
J: yeah
T: like that … and cakes like that … are just …
J: yeah
T: a tiny bit dear
J: yeah

It appears from this extract that J favours the use of *yeah* and *mm* as an interjection. He has used *yeah* eight times and *mm* twice. Of course, J has the option of using any number of different types of interjection, such as *uh huh*, *mm hm* and *oh*, but he restricts himself to just two in this extract. This repetitive use of *mm* and *yeah* has the effect of acknowledging the speaker's ongoing talk and of signalling that J is still attending to it.

Phonology

Phonological variation refers to the ways in which particular speech sounds may be altered in the spoken word, according to the geographical and/or social environment. Consider, for example, the pronunciation of the word *scone*. In England there are two main ways of pronouncing the vowel in this word. It may be short, as in the words c*o*n, h*o*t and l*o*ck, or it may be long, as in the words c*o*ne, l*ow* and s*o*. The selection and use of either the short or long vowel varies by geographical region. So, for example, the short vowel version of *scone* is generally favoured in the Tyneside area of the north-east, whereas the long vowel is the predominant form in Devonshire within the south-west. In addition to such geographical differences, vowel selection is also influenced by social circumstances. Staying with our example of *scone*, we find that within the north-east Tees Valley area of England, the use of the short vowel is commonly associated with the working classes and the long vowel with the upper middle classes.[1] This situation is often reversed within the East Riding of Yorkshire, where the long vowel is associated with working class and the short vowel with middle class. The recognition that variations in language and speech are influenced by geography and social circumstance has led to the development of the field of sociolinguistics that specifically investigates these phenomena.

Conscious and Unconscious Variation

Some aspects of the social use of language and speech appear to be the product of conscious choices and others do not. For example, I may wish to impress my new, male boss and, therefore, make a conscious effort to call him *Sir*, or I may wish to appease a police officer and, therefore, refer to them deliberately as *Officer*. Such choices are based on my assumptions of the likely impact of choosing a particular linguistic form. I could, of course, be wrong. Perhaps my new boss considers that the use of *Sir* indicates that I am fawning, deferential and weak? Perhaps the police officer considers that I am being patronising? User choice, then, is based on the assumption that we share the same interpretations. Other aspects of language use do not appear to be so consciously controlled, however. One possible candidate is phonology. For example, how do you pronounce the following words?

last
past
grass
laugh
bath

Do you pronounce them with a long vowel, as in the word _car_? Or do you pronounce them with a short vowel, as in the word _pan_? In England, people who live in the south predominantly use the long vowel, whereas the short vowel is largely associated with the north. In addition, the long vowel is regularly associated with middle-class speakers and the short vowel with working-class speakers. Whether or not we would agree with this, the fact remains that listeners will make judgements about the speaker (eg, their geographical origin and their socio-economic status), based on linguistic markers such as vowel length.

Accommodation
Sociolinguistics has demonstrated that certain social groups vary features such as syntax, morphology, vocabulary and phonology in a systematically different way from other social groups. This observation leads to the concept of accommodation (Hudson, 1996). So, for example, if I wish to identify myself as a member of a particular social group (golf club, occupational group, Manchester United football supporters' group, etc), it is likely that I will accommodate the style of speaking promoted by that particular group. This tends to reinforce group cohesion and solidarity. My style of speaking will identify me as being in or outside the group. The converse of this will also operate, ie, if the group wishes actively to keep others at a distance and restrict access, the language and speech developed may be so esoteric that it is difficult, if not impossible, for outsiders to accommodate the style of speaking. In summary, the particular style of speaking, as identified by syntactic, morphological, lexical (ie, vocabulary) and phonological choices, is one of the strongest indicators of affiliation to a particular social group.

Time-limited Variation

Variations in syntax, morphology, vocabulary and phonology are often time-limited, ie, certain words, phrases, clause constructions and pronunciations are popular only for a particular period of time. For example, *bus* is now commonly taught as a vocabulary item to foreigners learning the prescriptive English grammar. However, it is derived from the now less frequently used word *omnibus*. Similarly, *pram* is used for the older term *perambulator*. It is these sorts of variations that allow us to judge an utterance, or written sentence, as being either contemporary or dated. Take a look at the humorous cartoons 'Miffy' and 'CyberPunk'.

If you are able to ignore the stylised drawing of each cartoon and focus just on the language it should be obvious that 'Miffy', with phrases such as *fearfully bucked* and *thrashed him within an inch of his life*, is somewhat older than the more contemporary 'CyberPunk'. Such phrases do not generally appear within the current common vernacular. In fact, 'Miffy' was first published in 1923. In contrast, 'CyberPunk' incorporates a very different set of vocabulary items and phrases. For example, the noun *android*, the noun modifier *terrabyte* and the phrase *software architecture* set it apart from the time period of 'Miffy', and squarely within the popular culture of the present or even future time. In addition, 'CyberPunk' includes a number of neologisms, ie, invented words or meanings, such as the verbs *gunned* and *jacked-in*. These items contribute to the contemporary, or futuristic, milieu. A final point relating to the 'Miffy' cartoon is that the subject matter is of a man telling a joke about his wife. Such a theme is now likely to be considered politically incorrect within the United Kingdom. That is to say, wives, mothers-in-law, people with disabilities, and members of ethnic minority groups, for example, are no longer considered appropriate targets for certain kinds of joke. The point to be made here is that we will also make judgements about the historical placement of a spoken or written text based on its thematic content. However, whereas morphology, syntax, vocabulary and phonology, are linguistic in nature, content is not. In other words, we can make linguistic choices about how to vary morphology, syntax, vocabulary and phonology but we cannot make a specifically linguistic choice over the selection of content: we apply whatever linguistic features we choose to any selected content.

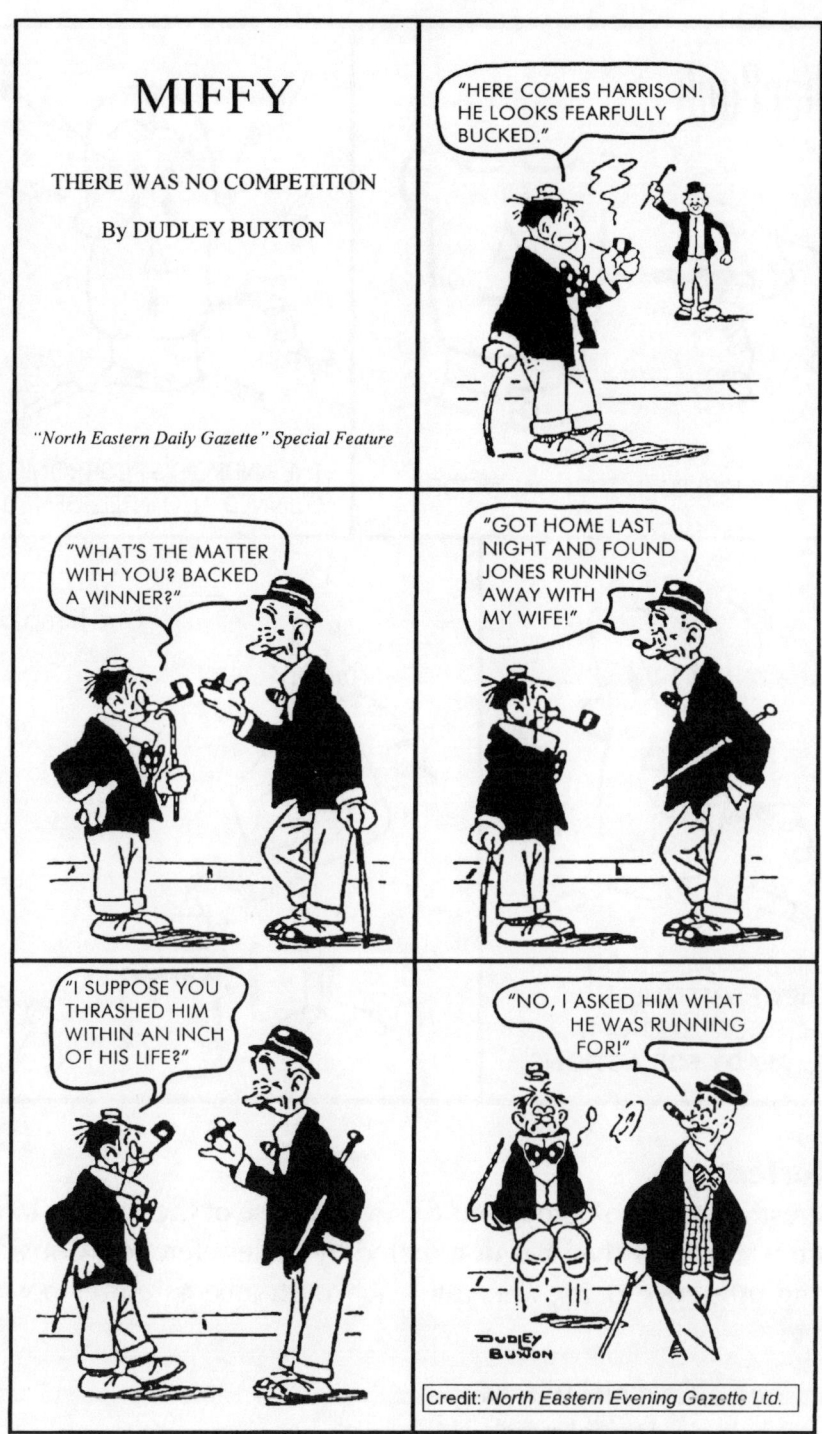

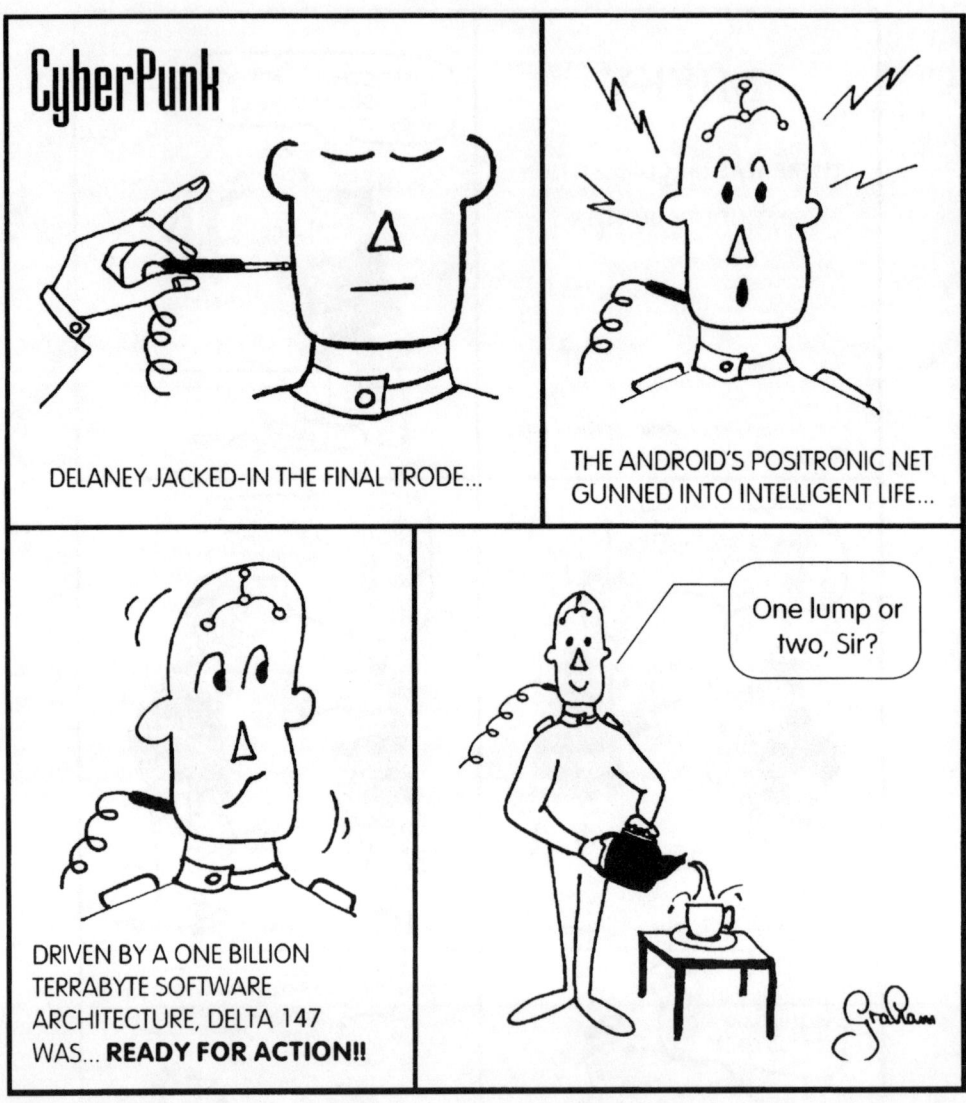

Genderlect

An interesting point to note about the general use of the English language in western society is that it is dominated by male reference. Consider the following utterance pairs, and rate each utterance as either positive or negative:

A   he's a financial wizard
B   she's a financial witch

A   he's a proper courtier
B   she's a proper courtesan

A   you big boy's shirt
B   you big girl's blouse

Generally, people perceive the A utterances as positive and the B utterances as negative. But what is the difference between them? The only significant difference is that the A utterances use a male vocabulary item and the B utterances use a parallel female vocabulary item. For example, a *wizard* is a male sorcerer and a *witch* his female counterpart. Note how the male term is used to suggest something positive, ie, being a financial wizard suggests that the person is a highly skilled and successful accountant. However, to say, *she's a financial witch* is to suggest that the person is an incompetent accountant. Similarly, the somewhat dated terms *courtier* and *courtesan* were once used to indicate a male and female attendant at a royal court respectively. Nowadays, it is the female term that is used in derogatory fashion to suggest that someone is a whore or prostitute. The male term continues to propose a rather charming individual who courts favour by flattery. Again, it is the female reference that is promoted as the negative and debased term. While *witch* and *courtesan* disparage the roles played by women, even women's dress is not immune. In the UK the term *blouse* is usually reserved to refer to a loose-fitting garment which extends to the waist and which is worn by females. The analogous garment worn by men is referred to as a *shirt*. Once more, in the final pair of utterances it is utterance B, which uses the female vocabulary item, which is typically perceived to be derisory. In fact, utterance A is typically perceived as a witty restructuring of the derogatory utterance B and, therefore, it creates a humorous effect from this negative reference. This use of language to reflect power relations between the sexes is referred to as genderlect. Other examples include the tendency to refer to machines, especially cars and ships, as female, eg, *She's running well* (meaning, 'The car has no mechanical faults at the moment') and *God bless all who sail in her* (typically uttered by one in authority, male or female, when naming and, thereby, commissioning a new ship). Why should this be? One suggestion is that machines are tools to be used and manipulated for a man's own ends and, some would

155

argue, this similarly reflects men's attitude to women throughout history, ie, that they are things to be manipulated for a man's own ends. A further example derives from the debate between various Christian denominations during the 1990s. The dispute centred on whether or not God should be referred to solely as 'Father', or whether or not God is also female and, therefore, should be referred to as 'Mother'. This has culminated in the publication of several Bible translations that incorporate inclusive language, ie, language that does not distinguish God, or God's blessings, in terms of gender.

The end of this chapter concludes Part 2 of the book and our overview of language. We turn our attention in the next chapter to the second major aspect of human communication, speech.

Revision Exercises

5.1 Define a holophrase.

5.2 Identify the semantic categories (*agent, object, action, location*) in the following utterances, eg, *the boy* (*agent*) *kicked* (*action*) *the ball* (*object*):

> *ball go net*
> *hit spoon table*
> *drink juice*
> *mummy sing*
> *eat dinner*
> *daddy dig garden*

5.3 What is the difference between slang and jargon?

Activities

5.4 For a full week keep a notebook in which you record any examples of genderlect. Note the gender of the person using genderlect. Do only males disparage females or do females also use language to disparage other females? Similarly, do females use any gender-specific terms to disparage males? Reflect on whether or not such terms make you feel uneasy. Why?

5.5 Choose two professions known to you, and either interview a member of each profession or consult 'trade' journals of the professions. Construct a list of jargon words and their meanings that are specific to that profession. How do these words promote efficient and effective communication between members of the same profession? Would the jargon words of the first chosen profession be readily understood by members of the second chosen profession?

Note

1 *Some readers may be uncomfortable with the use of labels such as 'working class' and 'middle class', considering such distinctions anathema in a modern society. However, these broad classifications are still assigned by the Registrar General's Office and they are used in much contemporary sociological research.*

CHAPTER 6

Speech Sounds

THIS CHAPTER INTRODUCES PART 3 of the book and begins our inquiry into speech. We start by setting out several definitions of speech as the primary transmission system of language. Subsequently, we discuss the differences between an orthographic and phonemic representation of speech sounds in written form, highlighting the weakness of normal writing methods and the strength of phonemic transcription. This discussion leads us to a definition of a phoneme as the simplest speech sound element that may be used to differentiate between one word and another. Next we introduce the first of the two types of speech sound, vowels. Vowels are described as 'open' sounds that are differentiated by differences in relation to shape of the lips, position of the tongue and jaws, and the length of vocalisation. Simple and complex vowels are also described. Subsequently, the bulk of the chapter is devoted to a description of the second class of speech sounds, consonants. Consonants are described as 'closed' sounds and space is devoted to an explanation of the articulation of five types: plosives, nasals, fricatives, affricates and approximants. Following this description a summary of the method for describing consonant sounds is given in relation to voicing, place of articulation and manner of articulation. Next, a distinction is made between a phoneme and other phonetic realisations of the same phoneme. The phonetic variation in these so-called allophones is outlined in relation to the concepts of aspiration, velarisation, de-voicing, dentalisation and nasalisation. This leads finally to a reconsideration of the method used for transcribing speech sounds and the notion of a broad or narrow transcription.

What is Speech?

As with our attempts to define language in Chapter 2, it is also difficult to come up with one overarching, all-inclusive, definition of *speech*. The definitions found in the literature vary from researcher to researcher, and they typically reflect the investigator's particular approach to the subject. For example, a researcher who is especially interested in the physics of sound is likely to propose a definition that focuses on the biomechanical and acoustic aspects of speech:

Speech is the sounds produced by alterations of the vocal apparatus to shape air expelled from the lungs.

One who is interested in meaning may well emphasise the ways in which particular speech sounds are used systematically to signal meaning in a language:

Speech is the sounds produced by the coordinated use of the voice and articulation to construct words that convey meaning, ie, the sounds of a particular language.

An investigator who is concerned with the variety of ways in which living organisms communicate may consider that:

Speech is the primary medium by which human beings communicate through language.

People interested in general human behaviour may note that:

Speech is a learnt system of communication.

All of these definitions are, of course, correct but no one definition captures the entire essence of what is meant by speech. Most of us, however, probably feel that we know intuitively what is meant by speech.

After all, we all speak, don't we? Isn't it one of the most natural things humans do? For most people speaking comes naturally, and yet it is a process that the majority of us are unable to explain. If you were asked to describe how you produce the sound /r/, as in the word r̲abbit, would you be able to do so? It is not such a simple matter. Most researchers divide the study of speech into two sub-fields. The first is phonetics. This sub-field is concerned with the sounds of particular languages and, principally, how these sounds are articulated. The second sub-field is phonology. A study of phonology concentrates on the specific ways in which the speech sounds are used in particular languages and, especially, the rules that govern their use. This chapter is concerned with phonetics and the area of phonology will be taken up in the following chapter. Before we begin our exploration of the articulation of English speech sounds, however, we will first consider a suitable methodology for representing speech sounds in written form.

Orthography and Phonemic Transcription
Consider the following:

> Daniel gave Kathryn a bow

What do you think was actually given? Did Daniel stand tall, half raise his right arm, pass it across his torso, smile at Kathryn, and then bend forward at the waist for a couple of seconds before standing upright again? Or did Daniel hand Kathryn a silk ribbon tied into a decorative knot? The problem in interpreting the above text is that we are relying solely on standard English writing, or orthography. Clearly, if we just write the word *bow*, you will not know if the word means 'to stoop' or 'a decorative knot'.[1] The difficulty lies in the fact that there is no one-to-one relationship between the alphabetic letters used in writing words and the actual sounds that make up those words when spoken. In English there are 26 letters in the alphabet, but there are approximately 44 speech sounds. In the case of *bow* it is the vowel that differs. If the word is used to mean bending or stooping then the vowel, in the spoken word, is the same as that in the words n̲ow̲, and c̲ow̲. If, however, we mean a decorative knot then a different vowel is spoken, this time it is the same sound as in the words sh̲ow̲, l̲ow̲, and kn̲ow̲. So, we say that the same orthographic representation can have a different acoustic representation. Consider the following list of words, all of which contain the alphabetic letter 'a'. Try and determine how many different sounds the letter 'a' represents:

act ace tall announcer animal ale late astride ball

There are actually four different sounds represented by the letter 'a' in the above examples:

act and _animal_ represent one sound (other examples include: _and_, _ant_, _pan_, _lamb_, _hamster_, _candle_)

ace, _ale_ and _late_ all have another sound the same (further examples include: _mate_, _Kate_, _date_, _lemonade_, _able_, _bane_)

tall and _ball_ share a third vowel sound (other examples include: _fall_, _hall_, _stalling_, _gall_, _caller_, _walled_)

announcer and _astride_ represent the fourth sound (it occurs in words such as: _astonish_, _arrange_, _abyss_, _annoy_, _astray_, _pasta_)

So, we see that in English the same alphabetic letter can represent different spoken sounds. Similarly, the same sound can be represented by different combinations of alphabetic letters. Consider the different spellings of the sound 'sh' in the following words:

ocean anxious condition fission fashion fuchsia

In addition to the above difficulties there are also 'silent' letters in English writing, ie, alphabetic letters that appear in the written word but which are never spoken. Examples include the 'k' in _knife_ and _knee_, and the 'b' in _limb_ and _doubt_. Clearly, then, English orthography is not a satisfactory way of transcribing English speech sounds. What is required is a system that has a direct one-to-one relationship between an actual sound and the symbol used to represent that sound. The system that is used is known as phonemic transcription. So, using the conventions of phonemic transcription, if we wished to indicate that the word _bow_ was intended to be pronounced with the same vowel sound as in the words _cow_ and _now_, we would transcribe it as /baʊ/, where /aʊ/ represents the vowel. If we intended to indicate that its pronunciation should be as in the words *no* and *sew*, then it would be transcribed as /bəʊ/ where, this time, /əʊ/ represents the different vowel. The simplest speech sound elements that are used to differentiate between one word and another are known as phonemes – hence the term 'phonemic transcription'. Phonemes are the counterpart element to morphemes: morphemes represent the smallest element of meaning in relation to language, and phonemes represent the smallest element of meaning in relation to speech. The word *bow* is actually made up of two phonemes, the consonant /b/ and either the vowel /əʊ/ or the vowel /ɑʊ/. We recognise the vowels as separate phonemes because they may be substituted in a word and, thereby, alter the meaning of the word. For example, /bɑʊ/ means 'to stoop', whereas /bəʊ/ means 'a decorative knot'. Similarly, consonants may be considered phonemes if they can also be substituted in words and, thereby, change the meaning of the word. For example, the initial consonant /b/ in the word /bəʊ/ *bow* may be substituted by the consonant /n/ to form the new word /nəʊ/ *no*. Throughout this book we will use the convention of enclosing phonemic representations of words within slanting lines, for example /dɪg/ *dig* and /kæt/ *cat*. The symbols used to represent each of the English phonemes will be those proposed by the International Phonetic Association (1999).

Vowels

Because we live in a literate society, most people think of vowels as being the five letters A, E, I, O and U. While this may be applicable to a discussion of reading and writing, in speech we recognise more than these. In fact, in English speech there are approximately 20 vowels. Vowels are described as 'open' sounds because they involve no obstruction to the flow of air from the lungs as it passes up through the trachea, through the larynx and out of the mouth. Other than a speaker positioning the tongue, jaws and lips in a specific configuration, there is nothing to obstruct the airflow. How, then, is one vowel distinguished from another? A full description of the production of vowel sounds is complicated and is beyond the scope of this book. However, in brief, a distinction is made between vowels dependent upon four main parameters that influence the shape of the oral cavity. They are (1) the shape of the lips, (2) the position of the tongue, (3) the position of the jaws, and (4) the length of the vocalisation. Each of these is outlined below.

Shape of the Lips

During the production of English vowels, just two lip shapes are normally adopted: (1) spread, and (2) rounded. This may be illustrated by alternating between saying the vowel sounds /i/, as in the word _eel_, and /u/, as in the word _shoe_. Look at yourself in a mirror as you alternate between saying these vowels aloud in rapid succession (/i/ – /u/ – /i/ – /u/ – /i/ – /u/). You will see that the lips are spread for the production of /i/, but that they are rounded and pushed forwards for the vowel /u/.

Position of the Tongue

The tongue can take up a variety of positions in the mouth during the production of vowels. The most obvious positions are: (1) a high position, where the tongue is raised towards the roof of the mouth, and (2) a low position, where the tongue is held close to the floor of the mouth. An example of the tongue occupying a high position is again the vowel sound /i/, as in the word _eel_. Try saying this sound aloud while looking in a mirror and both see and feel that the front portion of the tongue is elevated relatively high in the mouth. Now contrast this with the vowel /æ/, as in the word _ant_. This time you should notice that the tongue takes up a low position in the mouth.

Position of the Jaws

Vowels also differ from one another according to the extent to which the jaws are either (1) open, or (2) close (not 'closed', as a complete closure would prevent the free flow of air out of the mouth). Once again, look at yourself in a mirror and this time say the vowel sound /ɑ/, as in the word _art_. It should be obvious that the jaws are wide apart and you have adopted a relatively open mouth posture. Therefore this is an open vowel. Now contrast this with the vowel /i/, as in the word _eel_. This time, you should notice that not only is the tongue high and the lips spread, but that the jaw is close. Again, you can both see and feel the relative openness or closeness of the jaws by alternating the production of these vowels in quick succession (/i/ – /ɑ/ – /i/ – /ɑ/ – /i/ – /ɑ/).

Length of Vocalisation

Without exception, vowels are produced with the vocal folds vibrating. Therefore they are said to be voiced. In addition, vowels may be sustained for relatively longer and shorter intervals of time, ie, they are either (1) long, or (2) short. Try saying the vowel sound /ɔ/, as in the word p*or*t. This can be heard to be a relatively long vowel if you now contrast this by saying the vowel /ɒ/, as in p*o*t. A further example of a long vowel is /i/, as in p*ea*t. This can be contrasted with the short vowel /ɪ/, as in p*i*t. Again, try speaking aloud these two words, alternating between them, ie, *peat – pit – peat – pit*, and so on. This should help you distinguish the relative difference in the length of vocalisation of /i/ and /ɪ/.

Simple Vowels

When the speaker assumes only a single configuration of the lips, tongue and jaws – ie, there is no movement of these articulators during production of the vowel – then the speaker produces what is known as a simple vowel. There are 12 of these in English. Examples include, /ɒ/ as in p*o*t, /ʊ/ as in p*u*t and /æ/ as in b*a*t. Try saying these vowel sounds on their own. You should notice that once you have set the right position for your lips, tongue and jaws this does not alter in any way while you are producing the sound. Owing to this single configuration of the oral cavity, simple vowels are often referred to as monophthongs. The 12 English monophthongs are summarised in Table 6.1.

Complex Vowels

Some vowels involve two changes in the configuration of the oral cavity during production of the sound. These are known as complex vowels and there are approximately eight of them, examples of which include /ɒɪ/ as in b*oy* and /ɑʊ/ as in n*ow*. Again, try saying these vowels on their own. This time, especially if you exaggerate your articulation, you should notice that your mouth shape changes as you produce these vowels. Complex vowels involving two changes in the configuration of the oral cavity are known as diphthongs. These are summarised in Table 6.2.

Table 6.1 *English Monophthongs*

no	symbol	example words
1	i	*bee sea meal bean*
2	ɪ	*ship lip hit myth*
3	ɛ	*bed said leapt any*
4	æ	*cat pan had ant*
5	ɜ	*burn worm turn bird*
6	ə	*astray agree cupboard annoy*
7	ʌ	*cut bung won some*
8	u	*shoe sue lunar boot*
9	ʊ	*put should look wood*
10	ɔ	*order law caught ball*
11	ɒ	*pot hot long watch*
12	ɑ	*arm half car heart*

Table 6.2 *English Diphthongs*

no	symbol	example words
1	ɪə	*queer here near fear*
2	ɛə	*square there stair lair*
3	ʊə	*doer newer lure manure*
4	eɪ	*daily make lay cradle*
5	aɪ	*my try sigh eye*
6	ɒɪ	*noise boy boil oyster*
7	əʊ	*know toe owe photon*
8	ɑʊ	*now trout cow bough*

The Number of English Vowels

Recall that earlier we noted that there are *approximately* 20 English vowels. Why were we not more precise? Surely there are 20 vowels or there are not? The reason we cannot be exact is that that there is a great deal of variation in the way people produce vowel sounds. The vowels that we have been describing in this chapter are those that are commonly used in southern British English. Consequently, depending upon your own accent, you may or may not have agreed with the choice of words used to exemplify the various vowel sounds. For example, for many people living in the south of England the word *one* is pronounced /wʌn/, being pronounced exactly the same as the word *won*. That is to say, for these speakers, *one* and *won* are homophones, ie, the words have the same pronunciation but they have different meanings. In contrast, for a large number of speakers who live in the north of England the word *one* is pronounced /wɒn/, while *won* is pronounced as /wʊn/. Thus, for these speakers, the two words are not homophones, ie, they do not sound the same. Similarly, some accents use a monophthong where others use a diphthong. For example, rather than pronouncing words such as *poor* and *tour* with the diphthong /ʊə/, these words may be realised by the use of the monophthong /ɔ/, ie, /pɔ/and /tɔ/ instead of /pʊə/ and /tʊə/. While a full description of accents is beyond the scope of this book, we can note that it is mainly the quality of the vowels that are used that defines a person's regional accent.

Consonants

Recall that we describe vowels as 'open' sounds because there is no obstruction to the flow of air as it passes out of the mouth. In contrast, consonants are 'closed' sounds. This means that there is some type of obstruction to the airflow from the lungs by parts of the mouth coming into contact with each other, or very nearly contacting, thus closing off the free flow of air. For example, the lips could come together for the sound /b/ as in *ball*, or the tongue tip could almost contact the alveolar ridge just behind the upper incisors for the sound /s/ as in *sun*. These contacts, and near contacts, impede the free flow of air through the vocal apparatus. It is this kind of closure that characterises consonant sounds. In English there are approximately 24 consonants, and these are arranged into five main groups: (1) plosives, (2) nasals, (3) fricatives, (4) affricates, and (5) approximants. We will consider each of these in turn.

Plosives

Plosive consonants are oral sounds, ie, the soft palate is raised so that air from the lungs cannot pass upwards into the nasal cavity. Therefore, the air can only escape through the oral cavity. All plosives are produced by a complete obstruction of the airflow at some position in the mouth, for example by the lips coming together. Air from the lungs is then compressed behind the temporary obstruction and the air pressure builds up in the mouth. The obstruction is then rapidly removed (in this case, by the lips parting), and the air rushes out of the mouth with a slight 'explosion', hence the name *plosive*. Because plosives are made by a complete obstruction that briefly stops the airflow, they may also be referred to as *stops*. Plosives, or stops, occur in pairs and may be produced with or without the vocal folds vibrating. Recall that sounds produced without vocal fold vibration are said to be voiceless and those produced with vocal fold vibration are said to be voiced. There are three pairs of voiceless-voiced plosives. These are outlined below.

Bilabial Plosives

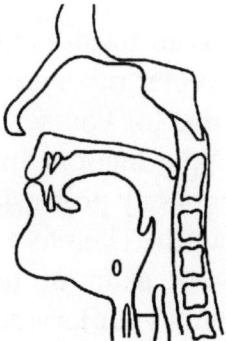

Figure 6.1 *Formation of Bilabial Plosives*

The first pair of plosive sounds are produced with the two lips coming together to form a complete closure, and they are known as bilabials, ie, two lips (see Figure 6.1). They are /p/, as in *pit*, *pan* and *cop*, and /b/, as in *bit*, *ban* and *lab*. You can test for yourself the effect of the voicing.

Hold your larynx gently but firmly between the index finger and thumb of one hand and say the sound /p/. Remember to say it as it sounds at the start of the word *pit* and not as the name of the alphabet letter, which would sound like /pi/. You should be unable to detect any changes in sensation through your fingers. Now say the sound /b/. You should feel a slight tingling sensation in your fingers as the vocal folds vibrate. The only difference, therefore, between /p/ and /b/ is that /b/ is voiced and /p/ is not. The developing child usually consolidates the use of bilabial plosives between 1;06 and 2;00 years of age.

Alveolar Plosives

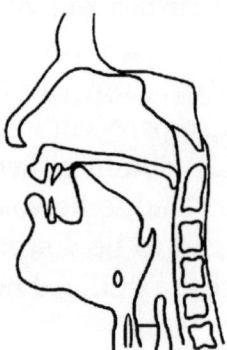

Figure 6.2 *Formation of Alveolar Plosives*

The second pair of voiceless-voiced plosives are articulated with the tip of the tongue contacting the alveolar ridge just behind the upper incisors (see Figure 6.2). You can feel this for yourself if you run the tip of your tongue backwards from your upper incisors and up over the roof of your mouth. The alveolar ridge is that bony protrusion just behind where your teeth meet the roof of your mouth. Therefore the sounds are known as alveolar plosives and they are /t/, as in *tin*, *tea* and *hat*, and /d/, as in *din*, *do* and *had*. Again, by holding your larynx as you say the sounds /t/ and /d/ you should notice a slight vibration in the larynx on production of /d/ but none when you produce /t/. This is because the vocal folds vibrate for /d/ but not for /t/. Therefore the alveolar plosive /d/ is voiced, and the alveolar plosive /t/ is voiceless. As with bilabial plosives, the developing child usually consolidates the use of alveolar plosives between 1;06 and 2;00 years of age.

Velar Plosives

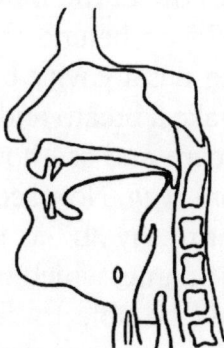

Figure 6.3 *Formation of Velar Plosives*

The third, and final, pair of plosive sounds are made with the back of the tongue contacting the soft palate or velum (see Figure 6.3). Therefore they are known as velar plosives. They consist of the sounds /k/, as in c̲oat, k̲ey and loc̲k̲, and /g/, as in g̲oat, g̲un and log̲. The velar plosive /k/ is voiceless and the velar plosive /g/ is voiced. The velar plosives take a little longer for the developing child to acquire, typically emerging between 2;00 and 2;06 years, but they may not be fully consolidated until 2;06–3;00 years of age.

Summary of Plosive Consonants

Table 6.3 *English Plosives*

	voiceless	voiced
bilabial	p	b
alveolar	t	d
velar	k	g

Nasals

As described above, when a person makes any plosive sound, the soft palate is raised so that it touches the back of the throat above the pharynx. This prevents air escaping through the nose, so all air is directed out through the mouth. All consonants produced in this way are referred to as oral consonants. Nasal sounds are similar to plosives in that there is a complete obstruction of the airflow in the mouth but, in contrast, the air pressure is not allowed to build up behind the obstruction. Rather, it is allowed to escape through the nasal cavity by lowering the soft palate. Consequently, it is possible to take a breath and prolong a nasal sound. Try it for yourself. Take a deep breath and see how long you can sustain the nasal sound /m/, as in the word _man_. Now see how long you can support a /b/ sound. Again, remember to say /b/ as it sounds at the start of the word _bin_ and not its alphabetic name, which would sound like /bi/. With a good breath an adult should be able to sustain /m/ for at least 10 seconds but /b/, if articulated correctly, can not be held for more than a brief instant: the air escapes and that is the end of it. Therfore nasals are continuant sounds because there is a continuous passage of the air stream through the vocal apparatus. There are only three English nasal consonants and they are all voiced. They are made in exactly the same position in the mouth as the plosives, and so they are named similarly. As we have seen there are bilabial, alveolar, and velar plosives and, likewise, there are bilabial, alveolar and velar nasals.

Bilabial Nasal

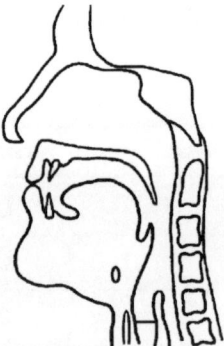

Figure 6.4 _Formation of Bilabial Nasal_

The nasal made furthest forward in the mouth is /m/, as in _mop_, _may_ and _ham_, and it is formed by the lips coming together to produce the obstruction (see Figure 6.4). As already mentioned, however, the air is allowed to escape continuously through the nose rather than exploding out through the mouth. The bilabial nasal is one of the first sounds to emerge in the developing child, and its use is typically consolidated between 1;06 and 2;00 years of age.

Alveolar Nasal

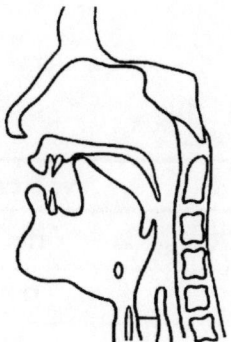

Figure 6.5 *Formation of Alveolar Nasal*

The next nasal back in the mouth is the sound /n/, as in <u>n</u>ot, <u>kn</u>ee and loa<u>n</u>. This is made with the obstruction between the tongue tip and alveolar ridge (see Figure 6.5), and it is, therefore, the alveolar nasal. As with the bilabial nasal, the alveolar nasal is also consolidated between 1;06 and 2;00 years.

Velar Nasal

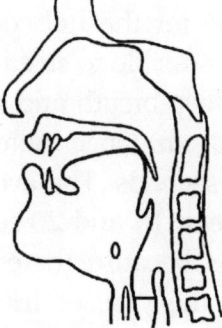

Figure 6.6 *Formation of Velar Nasal*

The third nasal, the furthest back in the mouth, is articulated by forming an obstruction by the back of the tongue contacting the velum (see Figure 6.6).

Therefore it is referred to as the velar nasal. This is the sound /ŋ/, as in the final sound of *sing*, *wing* and *ring*. This sound never appears at the beginning of words in English. The velar nasal, like velar plosives, emerges later than its bilabial and alveolar counterparts. It typically appears between 2;00 and 2;06 years, but may not be fully consolidated until 2;06–3;00 years.

Summary of Nasal Consonants

Table 6.4 *English Nasals*

	voiceless	voiced
bilabial	–	m
alveolar	–	n
velar	–	ŋ

Fricatives

Fricative consonants are formed by a narrowing of the mouth passage by two articulators, such as the lips, teeth, tongue or palate, coming into near contact. The air forcing its way through the narrow gap creates turbulence or friction, hence the name *fricative*. In general, fricatives emerge later than the plosive sounds. The earliest sound may arise at about 2;00–2;06 years, but the later developing sounds may not arise until around 4;06 years. Consequently, as well as generally emerging later than plosives, it also takes a much longer period of time for the full complement of fricatives to be acquired. Like the nasals, it is possible to sustain fricative sounds for several seconds. Again, try taking a deep breath and see how long you can sustain the sound /s/, as in the word *sun*. Once more, it is evident that the sound may be sustained for several seconds. The average adult should be able to sustain a /s/ sound for between 15 and 20 seconds. We noted earlier that nasals are continuant sounds because there is a continuous flow of air through the nasal cavity. In the case of fricatives there is a continuous passage of the air stream through the oral cavity, despite its near closure. The soft palate is raised and they are oral sounds. They also belong to the class of consonant sounds known as continuants. Like plosives, fricatives occur mainly in voiceless-voiced pairs. There are four of these pairs.

Labio-Dental Fricatives

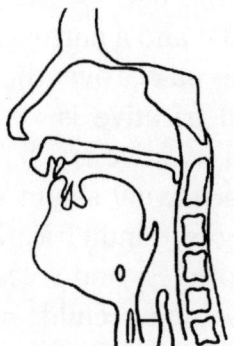

Figure 6.7 *Formation of Labio-Dental Fricatives*

The first pair of fricative sounds are articulated with a near contact of the bottom lip and upper incisors (see Figure 6.7). Friction is created as the air is forced between the lower lip and the upper incisors. So they are known as labio-dental fricatives. The two sounds are /f/, as in *fan*, *fish* and *half*, and /v/, as in *van*, *vote* and *rave*. The tongue lies relatively low in the mouth and it is not involved in the production of these consonants. The labio-dental fricative /f/ is voiceless and the labio-dental fricative /v/ is voiced. The voiceless labio-dental fricative usually emerges before the voiced labio-dental fricative, with /f/ emerging between 3;00 and 3;06 years, and /v/ emerging and becoming consolidated any time between 3;06 and 4;06 years.

Dental Fricatives

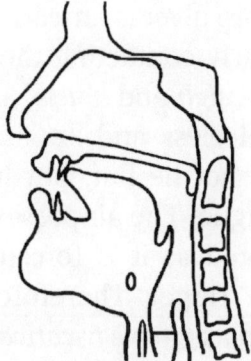

Figure 6.8 *Formation of Dental Fricatives*

The second pair of sounds are dental fricatives, and these are made by the tongue tip nearly contacting the back of the upper incisors (see Figure 6.8). The tongue is relatively flat and a narrow slit is formed in the mouth. The friction is created as the air passes over the tongue and past the upper incisors. The voiceless dental fricative is /θ/, as in *thin*, *thought* and *hearth*, and the voiced dental fricative is /ð/, as in *that*, *the* and *loathe*. Owing to the formation of a narrow slit in the mouth because of the relatively flat shape of the tongue, dental fricatives are sometimes referred to as *slit fricatives*. Both the voiceless and voiced dental fricatives are late emerging sounds in the developing child, and they are typically not consolidated until at least around 4;06 years of age.

Alveolar Fricatives

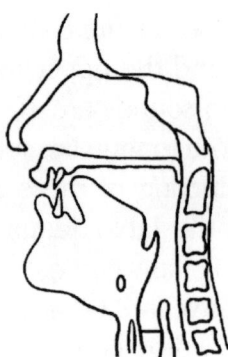

Figure 6.9 *Formation of Alveolar Fricatives*

The third pair of fricatives are alveolar fricatives, and they are formed by the front of the tongue nearly contacting the alveolar ridge (see Figure 6.9). They are /s/, as in *sun*, *sigh* and *house*, and /z/, as in *zoo*, *zebra* and *raise*. The sound /s/ is voiceless and /z/ is voiced. Unlike the dental fricatives, the tongue does not lie flat, but instead a groove is formed along the midline of the tongue. The air passes over the tongue along this groove and friction is created as it is forced between the front of the tongue and the alveolar ridge. Therefore, alveolar fricatives are, therefore, sometimes known as *groove fricatives*. There is controversy over when the voiceless alveolar fricative /s/ is consolidated. Some would argue that this happens as early as 3;00–3;06 years. However, there appears to be a wide variation in the acquisition of this sound, and some children still may not have fully consolidated the sound by 4;06 years. The voiced counterpart /z/ is generally recognised to emerge later than the voiceless sound, becoming consolidated between 3;06 and 4;06 years.

Post-Alveolar Fricatives

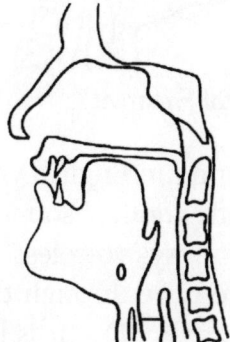

Figure 6.10 *Formation of Post-Alveolar Fricatives*

The final pair of fricatives are made somewhat further back in the mouth, with the middle of the tongue coming into near contact with the palate, just behind the alveolar ridge (see Figure 6.10). They are known as post-alveolar fricatives (meaning 'behind the alveolar ridge'), and they are /ʃ/, as in <u>sh</u>op, and /ʒ/, as in the middle sound of *mea<u>s</u>ure*. While the voiceless /ʃ/ can occur at the beginning, middle or end of words in English – eg <u>sh</u>oe, la<u>sh</u>ing and ma<u>sh</u> – the voiced /ʒ/ can never appear at the beginning of a word in English. This sound appears only in the middle and at the end of words, as in *vi<u>s</u>ion*, and in some pronunciations of *gara<u>g</u>e*. The voiceless post-alveolar fricative /ʃ/ emerges at any time between 3;06 and 4;06 years, and the voiced post-alveolar fricative /ʒ/ is usually not consolidated until the child is almost 4;06 years of age.

Glottal Fricative

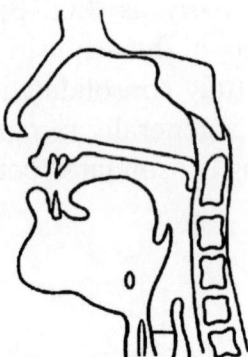

Figure 6.11 *Formation of Glottal Fricative*

There is one more fricative sound in English which is distinguished on the basis that it does not pair with another sound. It is the sound /h/, as in *house*, *hen* and *who*, and it is always voiceless. As it is made deep down in the throat by allowing air to escape through the chink between the vocal folds – ie, the glottis (see Figure 6.11) – it is known as a glottal fricative. Interestingly, the sound /h/ never appears at the ends of words in English. The glottal fricative is, in fact, the first fricative to emerge, and it can usually be identified in the speech of children between 2;00 and 2;06 years.

Summary of Fricative Consonants

Table 6.5 *English Fricatives*

	voiceless	voiced
labio-dental	f	v
dental	θ	ð
alveolar	s	z
post-alveolar	ʃ	ʒ
glottal	h	–

Affricates

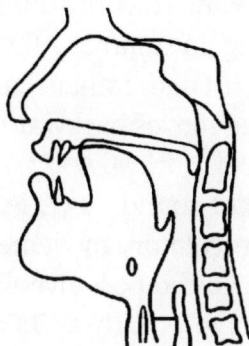

Figure 6.12 *Formation of Post-Alveolar Affricates*

All of the consonant sounds described so far are produced with either a complete obstruction of the airflow or a narrowing of the mouth passage. One pair of consonants, however, is produced by a combination of these two methods. These are the affricates. They begin with a complete obstruction formed by the tongue tip contacting the alveolar ridge, like alveolar plosives (see Figure 6.12). Then the air, instead of being released out of the mouth suddenly with an 'explosion', is released slowly with friction behind the alveolar ridge as the tongue moves backwards towards the palate. Consequently, they are known as post-alveolar affricates. The voiceless affricate is /tʃ/, as in <u>ch</u>ore, <u>ch</u>ain and ha<u>tch</u>. This is articulated first by the tongue tip contacting the alveolar ridge, as if to produce the voiceless plosive /t/. Then, instead of the air being released in a sudden 'explosion', it is released with friction as the tongue moves backwards in the mouth behind the alveolar ridge, as if to produce the voiceless post-alveolar fricative /ʃ/. This gives us the two-part sound /tʃ/. It is now possible to understand why the phonemic symbol for the voiceless post-alveolar affricate is written as /tʃ/. It is, of course, constructed from the two symbols that represent the two sounds that make up the consonant, ie, /t/ + /ʃ/ = /tʃ/. While it is possible to describe an affricate as a two-part sound, it is not heard as such. The speed of movement of the articulators is so great that it is heard as just one sound. Consequently, it is considered to be a single consonant. The voiceless affricate /tʃ/ usually arises at around the same time as the emergence of the voiceless post-alveolar fricative /ʃ/, ie, between 3;06 and 4;06 years.

The voiced counterpart affricate is /dʒ/, as in *jaw, jewel* and *large*, and this is assembled in a parallel way. The only difference this time, of course, is that the vocal folds are vibrating. In summary, the tongue rises as if to produce the voiced alveolar plosive /d/. Then, rather than an explosive release of air, friction is created as the tongue moves backwards towards the palate, as if to produce the voiced post-alveolar fricative /ʒ/. The combination of these movements creates the two-part sound /dʒ/, ie, /d/ + /ʒ/ = /dʒ/. Again, however, the rapidity of the articulatory movements means that it is heard as a single-sound consonant, the voiced post-alveolar fricative. Interestingly, the voiced affricate /dʒ/ may emerge as early as 3;06–4;06 years. Recall that the voiced post-alveolar fricative /ʒ/ is generally not consolidated until the child is about 4;06 years of age. This gives rise to a somewhat paradoxical situation. It appears that the developing child uses the voiced affricate, which incorporates the voiced post-alveolar fricative /ʒ/, before it uses the voiced post-alveolar fricative in its own right. A final brief point needs to be made. It should be apparent from the foregoing descriptions that affricates, being constructed from plosives and fricatives, are oral sounds and that, therefore, they are produced with a raised soft palate.

Summary of Affricate Consonants

Table 6.6 *English Affricates*

	voiceless	voiced
post-alveolar	tʃ	dʒ

Approximants
Our description of consonant sounds has highlighted the different ways in which the free passage of air through the vocal apparatus may be impeded. So far we have discussed just two types of closure. The first is complete closure and the second is near-closure. Plosives and nasals are both formed through a complete closure, but it is the way the air is allowed to escape out of the vocal apparatus that distinguishes between the two. In the case of plosives there is plosion after the complete obstruction is rapidly released. With nasals the soft palate is lowered and the air is allowed to escape continuously through the nose. Fricatives are

produced by a near closure of the oral cavity, and affricates are constructed from a dynamic combination of complete closure and near closure. However, these two types of closure (complete closure and near-closure) are not the only types of closure in English. There is a third type known as a *lateral*. Here, the tongue tip forms a complete closure but the air is allowed to escape over the sides of the tongue and out of the oral cavity. A fourth type is described as near closure without friction. Here, the vocal apparatus is not completely obstructed, as with plosives and nasals, nor is the airflow restricted to such an extent that friction is generated. Instead, two articulators approximate closely together and the air is allowed to escape through the oral cavity in a continuous stream. Sounds produced in this manner are often referred to as frictionless continuants. To complicate matters slightly, the English lateral and the frictionless continuants are frequently grouped together and referred to as approximants. This is the convention that we will use in this book. There are only four approximants in English and they are all voiced. They are also all produced with the soft palate raised and so they are oral sounds. The English approximants are described below.

Bilabial Approximant

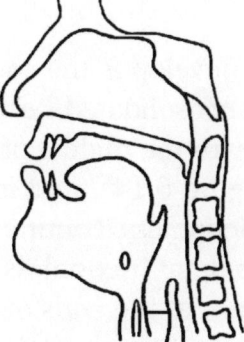

Figure 6.13 *Formation of Bilabial Approximant*

The first approximant to develop is /w/, as in the words <u>w</u>in, <u>w</u>hen and <u>w</u>e. It is usually established between the ages of 1;06 and 2;00 years. The sound is formed by the two lips approximating closely, but not so close that friction is generated (see Figure 6.13). The air stream then passes through this approximate closure and out of the mouth. This is the bilabial approximant or bilabial frictionless continuant. This sound may occur at the beginning of words such as <u>wh</u>y, <u>w</u>eek and <u>w</u>alk. However, it does not appear at the ends of words. The sound may be represented orthographically at the ends of words, for example in the word ho<u>w</u>, but it is not pronounced when speaking. In the case of *how*, this word is constructed from the voiceless glottal fricative /h/ plus the diphthong /aʊ/, ie, /haʊ/. It does not terminate with the bilabial approximant /w/.

Palatal Approximant

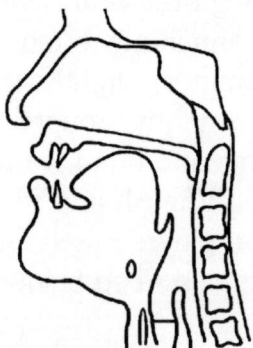

Figure 6.14 *Formation of Palatal Approximant*

The second approximant to develop is the sound /j/, as in <u>y</u>es, <u>y</u>ou and <u>y</u>ell. This sound is normally consolidated between the ages of 3;00 and 3;06 years. It is articulated with the middle of the tongue approximating closely to the palate (see Figure 6.14), and it is referred to as a palatal approximant, or palatal frictionless continuant. As with the bilabial frictionless continuant, the palatal frictionless continuant may appear at the beginning of words but not at the ends of words.

These first two approximants, the bilabial and the palatal, are commonly referred to as *glides*. Sometimes, however, they are described as *semi-vowels*. This is because the manner of their articulation is similar to particular monophthongs. The consonant /w/ is similar to the vowel /u/, as in b<u>oo</u>, sh<u>oe</u> and tw<u>o</u>, and the consonant /j/ is similar to the vowel /i/, as in b<u>ee</u>, f<u>eet</u> and kn<u>ee</u>. It is only because the two semi-vowels are arranged within syllables like other English consonants, and not like English vowels, that they are described as consonants (syllables are discussed in the next chapter).

Lateral Approximant

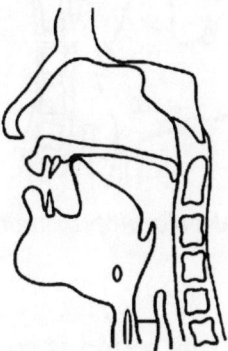

Figure 6.15 *Formation of Lateral Approximant*

The third approximant to arise in normally-developing speech is /l/, as in the words *love*, *lay* and *hall*. Typically, this appears any time between 3;00 and 4;06 years, but in some instances it may not be fully consolidated until around 6;00 years. The sound is a lateral. We noted earlier that a lateral is formed by the tongue tip forming a complete closure (see Figure 6.15) but instead of the air stream escaping over the tip of the tongue, the air spills over the sides of the tongue laterally. The point of closure for the sound /l/ is the alveolar ridge, and so it is known as an alveolar lateral approximant or, simply, the alveolar lateral.

Post-Alveolar Approximant

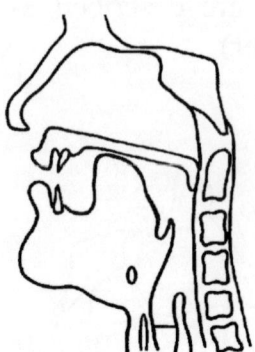

Figure 6.16 *Formation of Post-Alveolar Approximant*

The fourth, and final, approximant is /r/, as in <u>r</u>ed, <u>r</u>un and <u>r</u>ugby. The variation in the acquisition of this sound is considerable, being anything from 4;00 years up to 6;00 years in some instances. The sound is formed by the blade of the tongue approximating closely to a position just behind the alveolar ridge (see Figure 6.16). Consequently, it is known as the post-alveolar approximant, or post-alveolar frictionless continuant. It occurs at the beginning of words, but not at the end of words.

These latter two approximants, the lateral and post-alveolar approximants, are referred to as *liquids*.

The approximent consonants are summarised below in Table 6.7.

Summary of Approximant Consonants

Table 6.7 *English Approximants*

	voiceless	**voiced**
bilabial	–	w
post-alveolar	–	r
lateral	–	l
palatal	–	j

Voicing, Place and Manner of Articulation

During your reading of the above descriptions of English consonants you may have noted a pattern in the way each consonant sound is described. By convention each consonant is described in relation to three parameters, in the following order: (1) voicing, (2) place of articulation, and (3) manner of articulation.

Voicing

Voicing refers to whether or not the vocal folds are vibrating during the production of the consonant. If they are not vibrating the sound is voiceless, and if they are vibrating then the sound is voiced.

Place of Articulation

This refers to the place in the vocal apparatus where the two articulators come together. So, for example, bilabial means that the two lips come together, labio-dental means that the lower lip moves to make contact with the upper incisors, and alveolar means that the tongue tip moves towards the alveolar ridge. We have seen that there are eight places of articulation for English consonants: (1) bilabial, (2) labio-dental, (3) dental, (4) alveolar, (5) post-alveolar, (6) palatal, (7) velar, and (8) glottal. When two sounds have the same place of articulation they are said to be homorganic. For example, the oral sound /p/ and the nasal sound /m/ are both articulated with the lips, ie, they are bilabial. They are, therefore, homorganic. Similarly, the two sounds /s/ and /d/ are both articulated on the alveolar ridge. They too are homorganic.

Manner

This indicates the type of contact that is made between the two articulators. For example, the articulators could fully stop the flow of air out of the mouth before subsequently releasing it explosively, ie, a plosive. Another example is where the two articulators approximate closely, such that turbulence or friction is created, ie, a fricative. We have noted five possible manners of articulation in English: (1) plosive, (2) nasal, (3) fricative, (4) affricate, and (5) approximant.

Summary of English Consonants

From the foregoing discussion, we see that any consonant can be summarised in terms of a tripartite description that indicates its voicing, place of articulation and manner of articulation. For example, /p/ would be described as a voiceless bilabial plosive, /z/ as a voiced alveolar fricative, and /ŋ/ as a voiced velar nasal. Table 6.8 shows all the English consonants discussed so far (note that, conventionally, the voiceless phoneme is listed before its voiced counterpart).

Table 6.8 *English Consonants*

manner	place of articulation							
	bilabial	*labio-dental*	*dental*	*alveolar*	*post-alveolar*	*palatal*	*velar*	*glottal*
plosive	p b			t d			k g	
nasal	m			n			ŋ	
fricative		f v	θ ð	s z	ʃ ʒ			h
africative					tʃ dʒ			
approximant	w			l	r	j		

These consonant sounds are generally acquired in a front-to-back pattern, so that sounds made at the front of the mouth, such as /m/, /b/, and /p/, are used by the developing child before sounds made at the back of the mouth, such as /k/ and /g/. There are, of course, exceptions to this order. While we would generally expect a child to use the front sound /b/ before the back sound /k/, there will always be the child who does it the other way around. A suggested outline of the sequence of development of English speech sounds is presented in Table 6.9 but, as we have implied, the dates and pattern of acquisition are to be considered as guidelines only. It should be noted that it is not unusual for a child to be as old as 6;00–6;06 years of age before it may be fully capable of articulating all the speech sounds an adult would use.

Table 6.9 *The Order of Acquisition of English Consonants*

age (years)	new consonants used
1;06–2;00	m n p b t d w
2;00–2;06	k g ŋ h
2;06–3;06	f s j
3;06–4;06	v z l ʃ tʃ dʒ
4;06+	ʒ θ ð r

Allophones

Recall that we have defined phonemes as the simplest sounds which may be used to differentiate between one word and another. Essentially, a phoneme is an element of meaning. Consider the word *mad*, which we would transcribe as /mæd/. We could substitute the consonant /m/ with a /b/ in order to make the new word *bad* /bæd/. Consequently, /b/ is a phoneme, as it represents a minimal element of sound that can be used to create a difference in meaning. By reversing the argument it can be seen that /m/ is also a phoneme, as it can substitute for the /b/ in *bad* /bæd/ to make the new word *mad* /mæd/. Similarly, /t/ is considered to be a phoneme because it can replace the initial consonant in the words *man* /mæn/, *can* /kæn/ and *pan* /pæn/, and alter the meaning to make the new word *tan* /tæn/. So, when we have been transcribing English speech sounds we have been using symbols to represent only those sounds that make a difference in meaning in the language. We have called this phonemic transcription. However, not all speech sounds actually make a difference to the meaning of a word.

Aspiration

Consider the word *pot*. How is the sound /p/ articulated in this word? Is it the same as in the word *spot*? Try it for yourself. Say both words aloud and see if you can detect any differences between the two. You may need to say the words several times in succession, and quite forcefully, in order to notice any potential difference. If you are uncertain as to whether or not there is a difference, hold a flimsy piece of paper so that it hangs down closely in front of your mouth and then say the words again. What happens now? This time when you say the word *pot* you should see the paper blow quickly away from your lips as the /p/ is articulated. However, when you say *spot* there should be little or no movement of the paper when the /p/ is produced. What this demonstrates is that the sound /p/ is, in fact, articulated differently in both words. In the word *pot* the /p/ is accompanied by a short puff of air, ie, the sound is aspirated. The /p/ in *spot*, however, is not aspirated. Thus, we would say that the phonetic realisation of the phoneme /p/ is different in the words *pot* and *spot*. If we represent these phonetic differences symbolically then the aspirated /p/ is displayed as [pʰ]. By convention, phonemic transcriptions are represented within slanting lines / /, and phonetic transcriptions are displayed within square brackets [ ]. So the non-aspirated /p/ is represented as [p]. However, whereas /p/ and /b/ are able to make distinctions in meaning in English, ie, they are phonemes, [pʰ] and [p] are not. There is no essential difference in meaning, for example, between the words [pɒt] and [pʰɒt], they are merely articulated slightly differently. The sound [pʰ], therefore, has no contrastive function. It is said to be an allophone of the phoneme /p/. In summary, the phoneme /p/ has at least two allophones, [p] and [pʰ], each occurring in different contexts. In fact, the allophone [p] only occurs after a /s/ in English, and the allophone [pʰ] occurs in all other contexts. A similar reasoning may be applied to the phoneme /t/. When this occurs after /s/, as in a word like *stop* /stɒp/, there is no accompanying aspiration. However, in a word like *top* /tɒp/ aspiration is present. In fact, like /p/, /t/ is aspirated in all positions except when it follows /s/. Therefore, /t/ has at least two allophones, [t] and [tʰ]. There are many allophones in English, far too many to review here, but a few more examples should serve to illustrate the phonetic variation in how particular phonemes are realised.

Velarisation

We have noted that the lateral /l/ is formed by the tongue tip creating a complete closure at the alveolar ridge, and the air stream being allowed to escape over the sides of the tongue laterally. This sound appears in words such as _look_ /lʊk/, _silly_ /sɪlɪ/ and _like_ /laɪk/. However, in certain contexts, the quality of the sound is quite different. Compare the sound of /l/ at the beginning of the word _let_ /lɛt/ and at the end of the word _tell_ /tɛl/. When the lateral appears at the end of a word, the body of the tongue is slightly flatter, as the back of the tongue is raised towards the velum (see Figure 6.17). Therefore the sound is said to be velarised. We represent this allophone symbolically as [ɫ]. This allophone typically occurs at the end of a word, eg, _ball_ /bɔl/ → [bɔɫ]², or before another consonant, eg, _bolt_ /bəʊlt/ → [bəʊɫtʰ]. We can conclude, therefore, that /l/ has at least two allophones, [l] and [ɫ].

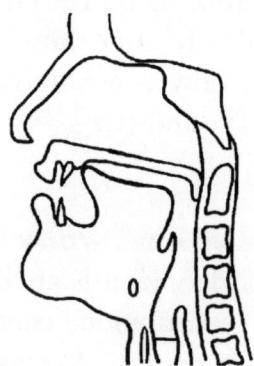

Figure 6.17 _Formation of Velarised /l/_

De-voicing

Consider how the phoneme /b/ is articulated in the word _bad_ /bæd/. You will probably need to say it aloud to both hear and feel the effect. Now try saying aloud the word _dab_ /dæb/, again focusing on the phoneme /b/. Do they sound the same? For most speakers, the /b/ at the beginning of the word _bad_ is fully voiced, ie, it is a strong sound. However, the /b/ at the end of the word _dab_ is typically less forceful, ie, it is not fully voiced. This phonetic realisation is referred to as being de-voiced and this de-voiced allophone of /b/ is represented symbolically as [b̥]. So we can say that /b/ has at least two allophones, [b] and [b̥].

There is also a de-voiced allophone of the phoneme /r/. This typically occurs after voiceless consonants such as /p/, /t/, /k/ and /f/, and it is represented symbolically as [ɹ̥]. It occurs in words such as _pray_ /preɪ/ → [pʰɹ̥eɪ], _train_ /treɪn/ → [tʰɹ̥eɪn], _crate_ /kreɪt/ → [kʰɹ̥eɪt], and friend /frɛnd/ → [fɹɛnd]. The fully voiced allophone is represented symbolically as [ɹ]. Thus, the phoneme /r/ has at least two allophones, [ɹ] and [ɹ̥].

We have noted that the lateral /l/ has at least two allophones, [l] and [ɫ]. In the same way that /b/ and /r/ may be de-voiced in certain contexts, /l/ may also be de-voiced. This typically occurs when the lateral immediately follows either the voiceless bilabial plosive /p/ or the voiceless velar plosive /k/. For example, in the word *play* /pleɪ/ it can be seen that the lateral follows on immediately after a voiceless bilabial plosive /p/. The lateral is consequently de-voiced and the word is realised as [pʰl̥eɪ]. Similarly, the lateral is de-voiced in the word *clay* /kleɪ/, in which it follows on immediately after the voiceless velar plosive /k/, ie, /kleɪ/ → [kʰl̥eɪ]. We must now conclude that the phoneme /l/ has at least three allophones, [l], [ɫ] and [l̥].

Dentalisation

We have seen how the plosive sound /d/ is articulated with the tongue tip contacting the alveolar ridge, ie, it is an alveolar plosive. While this is the predominant place of articulation, consider the placement of the tongue tip in the word *width* /wɪdθ/. In this instance, the tongue is not raised to the alveolar ridge, but is brought into contact with the back of the upper incisors. In other words, it is dentalised, being produced in the same place as the following dental fricative /θ/. This dentalised allophone of /d/ is represented as [d̪]. Consequently, the phoneme /d/ has at least two allophones – [d] and [d̪]. As well as the voiced alveolar /d/ becoming dentalised before a dental sound, the voiceless alveolar /t/ is similarly affected. For example, in the word *eighth* the alveolar assimilates the place of articulation of the immediately following dental fricative, and it becomes dentalised, represented symbolically as [t̪], ie, *eighth* /eɪtθ/ → [eɪt̪θ]. We must now recognise that the phoneme /t/ has at least three allophones, [t], [tʰ] and [t̪]. Other alveolars in similar contexts may also be dentalised. For example the alveolar nasal /n/ is dentalised in the word *plinth*, ie, /plɪnθ/ → [pʰlɪn̪θ], indicating at least two allophones of /n/, [n] and [n̪]. In reality, there are actually very few examples of English words that contain an alveolar immediately before a dental sound. However, this principle of the dentalisation of alveolars is a common feature of connected speech and it will be referred to again in the next chapter.

Returning once more to the lateral /l/, it is also possible to find instances when this phoneme is dentalised. In the same way that /d/ is dentalised when it appears before a dental fricative, /l/ is also dentalised in this context. Consider the following:

health   /hɛlθ/   →   [hɛl̪θ]

This example demonstrates the dentalisation of /l/ very well. However, we must also take account of the fact that the /l/ appears before a consonant. Consequently, the /l/ is also velarised. Therefore the complete representation of this allophonic variation is as follows:

health   /hɛlθ/   →   [hɛɫ̪θ]

We may now conclude that the phoneme /l/ has at least four allophones – [l], [ɫ], [l̪] and [ɫ̪]. In fact, this is the total number of allophones for this phoneme in English, no more are to be found.

Nasalisation

So far we have examined only allophones of consonants, but vowels are also subject to phonetic variations, depending upon the environment in which they occur. Consider the vowel /ɑ/ in the word *art* /ɑt/. Now listen to the difference in the quality of the same vowel in the word *mart* /mɑt/. In this instance, you may have been able to detect a slight nasal quality to the vowel. Rather than the air escaping fully through the mouth, as in the word *art* /ɑt/, the soft palate is lowered slightly such that some of the air escapes through the nose, giving it a nasal quality. The nasalised allophone of /ɑ/ is written as [ɑ̃]. The phoneme /ɑ/, therefore, has at least two allophones – [ɑ] and [ɑ̃]. This nasalisation of vowels typically occurs when the vowel immediately precedes, or follows, a nasal consonant, ie, /m/, /n/, /ŋ/, as in words such as *man* [mæ̃n], *now* [nɑ̃ʊ̃] and *wing* [wɪ̃ŋ]. Table 6.10 summarises all the allophones that have been discussed in this section.

Table 6.10 *Selected Allophones of English*

/p/	→	[p] after /s/ [pʰ] elsewhere
/b/	→	[b̥] in word-final position [b] elsewhere
/t/	→	[t] after /s/ [t̪] before /θ, ð/ [tʰ] elsewhere
/d/	→	[d̪] before /θ, ð/
/n/	→	[n̪] before /θ, ð/
/l/	→	[ɫ] before a consonant or in word-final position [l̥] after /p, k/ [l̪] before /θ, ð/ [l] elsewhere
/r/	→	[ɹ̥] before voiceless consonants
vowel	→	nasalised before or after /m, n, ŋ/

Narrow and Broad Transcription

It should be apparent, following our discussion of allophones, that speech sounds can be transcribed in two ways: phonetically or phonemically. A full phonetic transcription records all of the salient features of a sound's production, such as aspiration, de-voicing, dentalisation and nasalisation. This is sometimes confusingly referred to as a narrow transcription. Here, 'narrow' refers to the fineness of the detail that is recorded. Thus, the word *print* would be transcribed phonetically as [pʰɹ̥ɪ̃ntʰ]. We see that the voiceless alveolar plosive /p/ is aspirated, the post-alveolar approximant /r/ is de-voiced, the vowel /ɪ/ is nasalised, and the voiceless alveolar plosive /t/ is also aspirated. Therefore this narrow, phonetic transcription attempts to record all of the phonetic features of the spoken word. In contrast, if we were to transcribe *print* phonemically we would write it as /prɪnt/. Here we have made no attempt to record the phonetic variations. Rather, we have only recorded those features that make a difference to the meaning of words, ie, the phonemes. Consequently, phonemic transcription is sometimes referred to as a broad transcription. You will appreciate that the choice of transcription method is dependent upon one's purpose. If a narrow, detailed account of all phonetic features is required, then only a phonetic transcription will suffice. However, if it is sufficient merely to contrast larger meaning elements, then a phonemic transcription will be the favoured option.

This concludes our discussion of the phonetics of English. In the next chapter we consider how speech sounds are organised systematically. This is the second facet of speech, known as phonology.

Revision Exercises

6.1 Make a description of the following speech sounds as illustrated in the example, eg, the **p** of *pot* – voiceless bilabial plosive, the **z** of *zoo* – voiced alveolar fricative:

> the **tch** of *hutch*
> the **c** of *cat*
> the **ph** of *philosophy*
> the **se** of *nose*
> the **ng** of *wing*
> the **ll** of *yellow*
> the **m** of *mouse*

6.2 Transcribe the following words using the symbols of the International Phonetic Alphabet as set out in Tables 6.1, 6.2 and 6.8, eg, *bid* /bɪd/, *ten* /tɛn/, *throat* /θrəʊt/:

plant	*mood*	*zebra*	*jaw*
bird	*nose*	*thought*	*work*
talk	*ring*	*the*	*red*
dent	*fan*	*shop*	*lamp*
kiln	*vase*	*measure*	*yacht*
gravel	*sock*	*chop*	*house*

6.3 Make a broad (phonemic) and narrow (phonetic) transcription of the following words, noting any aspiration and nasalisation, eg, *pea* /pi/ [pʰi], *ban* /bæn/ [bæ̃n]:

pin
spin
pit
spit
Spain
map

Activities

6.4 Working with a partner, have your partner say aloud each of the monophthongs listed in Table 6.1. As you observe their production, try to describe each vowel in terms of (a) the shape of the lips, (b) position of the tongue, (c) position of the jaws, and (d) the length of the vocalisation. Present this information as a table.

6.5 Listen to a 3-year-old child at play with its peers. Make a phonemic inventory of consonants, ie, list all of the consonants that the child is able to produce. Is the child able to produce all of the English consonants or are there some gaps? Is there anything distinctive about the sounds that are not used? Can you explain the gaps in terms of the child's expected development?

Notes

1 *There are, of course, several other definitions of the word **bow**, eg, the front of a ship, a tool for playing the strings of a cello, a weapon for shooting arrows. However, for the purposes of the current argument it is convenient to ignore these other meanings.*

2 *We will also use the convention of an arrow (→) to signify 'is realised as'. Thus, /bɔl/ → [bɔt] is read as '/bɔl/ is realised as [bɔt]'.*

CHAPTER 7

The Speech Sound System

THIS CHAPTER INTRODUCES the field of phonology, ie, how speech sounds are systematically organised. First, three levels of organisation are considered: phonemic, syllabic, and word level. Consideration is then given to the notion of stressed and unstressed syllables. The majority of the chapter is dedicated to a discussion of phonological simplifying processes, ie, the various ways in which words may be reformulated through an alteration to their basic structure, or through other systematic changes, such as the substitution of speech sounds. The structural processes of deletion, cluster reduction, metathesis and epenthesis are described and exemplified. Following this, three types of systemic process are introduced: substitutions, assimilations and feature synthesis. The chapter is completed by demonstrating that phonological processes are not mutually exclusive, and that they may co-occur in the speech of any one individual.

Organisation of the Speech Sound System

We have seen that phonetics is concerned with how human beings articulate speech sounds through the coordinated use of the vocal apparatus. In contrast, phonology considers how specific sounds function systematically in a particular language. In short, phonology is concerned with a language's sound system. Specifically, it examines the organisation of speech units and considers how this transmits meaning. The sound system is organised at least at three levels: (1) phonemic, (2) syllabic, and (3) word. Each of these levels of speech sound organisation will be considered in turn.

Phonemic Organisation

We noted in Chapter 3 that morphemes are the smallest element of meaning in a language. Except for free morphemes, they are only meaningful when combined with other morphemes. For example, -ing on its own is meaningless. However, when combined with another morpheme, such as run, a new meaning is created, ie, running. The same is true of phonemes. On their own they are meaningless, eg, /t/, /l/ and /f/ spoken in isolation convey no meaning. It is only when they are combined that their contrastive function becomes evident, and that they are capable of signalling meaning. This combination of phonemes is the basic level of phonological organisation. The following examples indicate how the phonemes /t/, /l/ and /f/ may each be combined with the phoneme /i/ to produce different meanings:

$$/t/ \quad + \quad /i/ \quad = \quad /ti/ \quad tea$$
$$/l/ \quad + \quad /i/ \quad = \quad /li/ \quad Lee$$
$$/f/ \quad + \quad /i/ \quad = \quad /fi/ \quad fee$$

Organisation of Syllables

We see, then, how phonemes may be combined to form words. However, there is an intermediate level of phonological organisation known as the syllable. The most common form of syllable has a potential three-part structure, as follows:

C   V   C
consonant vowel consonant

The central vowel is referred to as the nucleus and, according to this potential structure, every syllable must consist of at least a nucleus, ie, a vowel sound. Examples include the following:

V	a	/eɪ/
V	I	/aɪ/
V	or	/ɔ/

Up to three consonants may be placed before the nucleus. This is known as the *prevocalic* position. Examples of syllables consisting of prevocalic consonant(s) plus a nuclear vowel include:

CV   *go*   /gəʊ/
CCV   *snow*   /snəʊ/
CCCV   *straw*   /strɔ/

In addition, up to four consonants may be arranged after the vowel. This is the *post-vocalic* position, and examples of syllables consisting of post-vocalic consonant(s) and a nuclear vowel include the following:

VC   *art*   /ɑt/
VCC   *arts*   /ɑts/
VCCC   *ants*   /ænts/
VCCCC   *(t)exts*   /(t)ɛksts/

As can be seen from the fourth example of *texts* above, consonants may occur in both prevocalic and post-vocalic positions within the same syllable. Further examples of this three-part structure include:

CCVC   *plane*   /pleɪn/
CCCVC   *splash*   /splæʃ/
CVCC   *malt*   /mɒlt/

Sequences of consonants such as these, in either prevocalic or post-vocalic position, are referred to as clusters (sometimes also known as *blends*). Therefore, the potential three-part structure of syllables may be summarised as follows:

        CCC   –   V   –   CCCC
    prevocalic   nucleus   post-vocalic

Syllabic Consonants
Consider the syllables that make up the following word:

    garden   /gɑ/ + /dən/ = /gɑdən/

The first syllable consists of a CV sequence and the second of a CVC arrangement. The first syllable is said to be a stressed syllable, ie, it is given more weight, more emphasis, when spoken. The first syllable is consequently given more prominence through this increased loudness. The second syllable is an unstressed syllable. In unstressed syllables that end in /n/ the immediately preceding vowel is usually the neutral vowel /ə/. Sometimes when words containing such syllables are spoken in connected speech, the neutral vowel is omitted altogether. This results in the final /n/ taking on the full measure of the syllable. This is known as *syllabic n* and it is transcribed as [n̩]. Thus:

garden /gɑdən/ → [gɑdn̩][1]

We see that the second syllable no longer contains a vowel. This is why we said earlier that the most common form of syllable has a potential three-part structure that consists minimally of a nuclear vowel. We see now that syllabic consonants are the exception to this rule. Further examples of *syllabic n* include the following:

frighten /fraɪtən/ → [fɹaɪtn̩]
button /bʌtən/ → [bʌtn̩]
Skipton /skɪptən/ → [skɪptn̩]

As well as the occurrence of *syllabic n* in unstressed syllables in word-final position, we also find a *syllabic l* appearing in the same position. Examples of *syllabic l*, which similarly take the full measure of a syllable, include the following:

handle /hændəl/ → [hændl̩]
bottle /bɒtəl/ → [bɒtl̩]
spangle /spæŋgəl/ → [spæŋgl̩]

Organisation of Words

As can be seen from the examples of syllables provided so far, the simplest words consist of just one syllable, ie, they are monosyllabic. We have seen how some words are constructed from just one nuclear vowel, eg, *a*, *I*, and *or*. Other monosyllabic words may consist of up to three prevocalic and four post-vocalic consonants. Consider the following that demonstrates the full compliment of prevocalic and post-vocalic consonants in one monosyllabic word:

CCCVCCCC *strengths* /strɛŋkθs/

Many words are, of course, constructed from more than one syllable, ie, they are polysyllabic. Whereas it is easy enough to define the number of prevocalic and post-vocalic consonants that may combine with a vowel to form a syllable, it is not as simple to define the maximum number of syllables that may combine to form a single word. The range is extremely wide. The smallest polysyllabic word is created from the combination of just two syllables, ie, they form a disyllabic word, eg, *garden, monkey, trumpet*. However, there are examples of words made up of three, four, five and more syllables. In the case of many technical words, such as the names of manufactured chemical compounds, there appears to be an almost endless concatenation of syllables, eg, *alpha-hydroxy-alpha-phenyl-benzeneacetic-acid-two-ethylpropylamino-ethyl ester* and *four-five-six-trihydroxy-seven-oxo-one-three-five-cycloheptatriene-one-two-dicarboxylic-anhydride*. However, this esoteric method of constructing names of chemical compounds is exceptional. Indeed, it follows its own rules of nomenclature as set out by the International Union of Pure and Applied Chemists (IUPAC, 1993). In comparison, the everyday, commonly spoken vocabulary of English does not appear to exceed about eight syllables per word. Some examples of everyday polysyllabic words are given below:

2 syllables: *furry*
/fɜ/ + /rɪ/ = /fɜrɪ/

3 syllables: *linguistic*
/lɪŋ/ + /gwɪs/ + /tɪk/ = /lɪŋgwɪstɪk/

4 syllables: *analysing*
/æn/ + /ə/ + /laɪ/ + /zɪŋ/ = /ænəlaɪzɪŋ/

5 syllables: *desensitising*
/di/ + /sɛn/ + /sə/ + /taɪz/ + /ɪŋ/ =
/disɛnsətaɪzɪŋ/

6 syllables: *uncharacteristic*
/ʌŋ/ + /kæ/ + /rək/ + /tə/ +/rɪs/ + /tɪk/ =
/ʌŋkærəktərɪstɪk/

7 syllables: *incompatibility*
/ɪŋ/ + /kəm/ + /pæt/ + /ə/ + /bɪl/ + /ə/ + /tɪ/
= /ɪŋkəmpætəbəlɪtɪ/

8 syllables: *internationalisation*
/ɪn/ + /tə/ + /næʃ/ +/ən/ + /əl/ + /aɪ/ +/zeɪ/ +
/ʃən/ = /ɪntənæʃənəlaɪzeɪʃən/

Stressed and Unstressed Syllables

We have already noted that some syllables in polysyllabic words may be given more emphasis than others, ie, they are stressed. This extra prominence is achieved predominantly, although not exclusively, by the speaker raising the pitch of the sounds that constitute the syllable. All English words have one syllable that receives primary stress. Many polysyllabic words also have another syllable that receives secondary stress. Syllables receiving secondary stress are still made prominent but less so than the syllable with primary stress. In contrast, some syllables receive no stress at all, ie, they are unstressed. We can signify primary stress by a superscript mark (') immediately before the affected syllable. Secondary stress may be indicated by a subscript mark (ˌ) immediately before the affected syllable, and unstressed syllables will be left unmarked. Consider the following polysyllabic word:

    programmer   /ˈprəʊˌgræmə/

The primary stress appears on the first syllable /ˈprəʊ/, the secondary stress on the second syllable /ˌgræm/ and the third, and final, syllable /ə/ is unstressed. However, not all English words pattern in this neat way: stress may fall on syllables in any position, for example:

    photograph   /ˈfəʊtəˌgrɑf/
    underpants   /ˌʌndəˈpænts/
    announcing   /əˈnaʊnˌsɪŋ/

Further, not every polysyllabic word has a secondary stress. Whereas the last example above – *announcing* – demonstrated primary and secondary stress together with an unstressed syllable, the word *announcer* has no secondary stress at all:

    announcer   /əˈnaʊnsə/

The mandatory primary stress is evident but, this time, the remaining two syllables are unstressed. Now consider the word *perfect* in the following example:

    a perfect life   /ə ˈpɜˌfɛkt ˈlaɪf/

Here, the disyllabic word *perfect* receives
syllable and secondary stress on the second s
with *perfect* in the following example:

> *to perfect life* /tʊ pəˈfɛkt ˈlaɪf/

In this instance, the primary stress is on the
is no secondary stress at all. It is apparent
functioning differently in each example, ie, they belong to different word
classes. The first *perfect* is an adjective and the second functions as a verb.
We see, then, how the placement of stress can exhibit a contrastive
function. However, unlike phonemes, which are always contrastive, stress
patterns may not always be so. Consider the word *profile* in the following:

> *a profile* /ə ˈprəʊˌfaɪl/
> *to profile* /tʊ ˈprəʊˌfaɪl/

The first use of *profile* is as a noun and the second as a verb. However,
in both instances the primary stress is placed on the first syllable and the
secondary stress on the second syllable. Therefore, stress alone is
insufficient to contrast these two uses of the word *profile*. This concludes
our discussion of the organisation of the speech sound system. Next we
turn our attention to phonological simplifying processes, ie, the different
ways in which words are reformulated through modifications of their
structure or other systematic alterations, such as the substitution of one
speech sound for another.

Phonological Simplifying Processes

Children below the age of about 4;06 years have not developed
sufficiently to fully coordinate the movement of their vocal apparatus. As
a consequence, certain sounds, sound combinations or transitions from
one sound to another are too difficult for them to perform. The child may,
therefore, use another sound that is simpler to produce, or restructure the
word, so that certain transitions are easier. But the child does not activate
these reformations randomly. There are certain rules, which are thought
to be genetically pre-programmed, which 'tell' it which of the simpler
sounds or sound combinations to use. However, the child is unaware of

₋ss of rule selection: it is an entirely unconscious act. Several of so-called phonological simplifying processes have been identified, ₋n one operating at a syllabic or word level. In order to illustrate how they might function in a normally developing speech sound system we will first consider an example of speech that is potentially disordered.

Speech Disorder

Suppose 4;00-year-old Adam is attempting to name a water bird related to geese and swans but, instead of producing the appropriate adult form /dʌk/, he says [dʌt]. What do you think is the problem? Do you suppose that Adam has difficulty in saying the voiceless velar plosive /k/? On a cursory inspection this appears to be a reasonable deduction. However, suppose I now inform you that Adam refers to the thing he drinks out of as a [kʌp]. Clearly, we have to revise our thinking because it is now apparent that Adam is, in fact, capable of saying the sound /k/ – in this case he is producing it in syllable-initial position. So why does he not produce it in syllable-final position, as in the word *duck* /dʌk/? The answer lies in the gross distinction that can be made between a phonetic disorder and a phonological disorder.

Phonetic Disorder

If a person is unable to articulate a particular speech sound then they will present a phonetic disorder (or articulation disorder). Recall from our earlier discussion of phonetics that each speech sound is the product of coordinated movements of the vocal apparatus used to interrupt or shape an egressive air stream from the lungs. There may be several physiological and/or anatomical impairments that prevent the proper articulation of speech sounds. These include cerebral palsy, cleft palate, and hearing impairment. In addition, because speech is a learnt skill, certain conditions that affect the learning process may interfere with a person's ability to articulate speech sounds. The most obvious example would be a general or specific learning disability, but psychological neuroses and psychoses may also have an effect. The simplest way to determine whether or not a person has a phonetic disorder is to conduct a stimulability test. This is fairly straightforward. Instruct the person as follows: 'Look at me and listen carefully. I'm going to say some sounds, and I want you to say them back to

me.' Then go through the whole repertoire of English con
saying them clearly one at a time. Make a note of whether or
was able to imitate the sound properly by placing a tick in tl
cell in Figure 7.1 or, if not, which sound (if any) they produce ... analysis
of this inventory will determine which consonants the person can articulate
and which they cannot. If the person is able to articulate a particular speech
sound then they cannot have a phonetic disorder with respect to that
particular sound. Only if the person cannot actually articulate a sound
would they be described as having an articulation difficulty.

sound	✔ (or sound produced)	sound	✔ (or sound produced)
p		z	
b		θ	
t		ð	
d		ʃ	
k		ʒ	
g		tʃ	
m		dʒ	
n		w	
ŋ		r	
f		l	
v		j	
s		h	

Figure 7.1 *Stimulability Test*

Phonological Disorder

Returning to our previous example of Adam referring to a *duck* as [dʌt],
we know that Adam cannot have a phonetic difficulty with respect to
articulating the sound /k/ because we know he can produce this sound

in the word *cup* /kʌp/. Let us have a better look at Adam's speech sound system. In Table 7.1 we list some further examples of how Adam says particular words. Study them for a moment and see if you can work out what is happening.

Table 7.1 *Sample of Adam's Speech*

no	word	realisation	no	word	realisation
1	cup	[kʌp]	9	pick	[pɪt]
2	gap	[gæp]	10	pig	[pɪd]
3	cut	[kʌt]	11	tuck	[tʌt]
4	got	[gɒt]	12	tag	[tæd]
5	cod	[kɒd]	13	duck	[dʌt]
6	God	[gɒd]	14	dig	[dɪd]
7	case	[keɪs]	15	sack	[sæt]
8	gas	[gæs]	16	sag	[sæd]

For the purpose of the current discussion we will ignore the vowels and concentrate solely on the consonants. What do you notice about the realisation of each of the consonants in words 1–8? Well, it is useful to consider first the structure of each word. You will notice that, if articulated correctly, each word should have a velar consonant in syllable-initial position, either /k/ or /g/. Further, only four consonants should appear in syllable-final position: /p/, /t/, /d/, or /s/. Finally, Adam does, in fact, realise each of the words as the appropriate adult form, ie, they are articulated correctly. This indicates that there is no specific phonetic difficulty with respect to articulating the sounds /k/, /g/, /p/, /t/, /d/ or /s/. Now examine words 9–16. Notice this time that in syllable-initial position there should be the same four consonants that appeared in syllable-final position in words 1–8, ie, /p/, /t/, /d/ or /s/. Again, Adam articulates these correctly. Now, note that each word, if articulated correctly, should have either /k/ or /g/ in syllable-final position. However, when we examine how Adam actually realises these words, it

is evident that he does not produce these velar conso.
Rather, he systematically substitutes [t] for /k/ and [d] for .
know that he can articulate these sounds correctly, we kno
be a phonetic error. Instead, because he is systematically   .₆ the
realisation of a particular set of consonants when they appear in a
particular position in words, he is said to have a phonological difficulty.
In this case, each syllable-final velar consonant is being substituted by an
alveolar consonant that is made further forwards in the mouth. Adam is,
in fact, demonstrating a phonological simplifying process known as
fronting. Before we can determine whether or not this is atypical and,
therefore, a speech disorder, we need to know if this process is a naturally
occurring process in a child aged 4;00 years. In the next sections we will
consider two categories of phonological simplifying process: (1)
structural simplifications, and (2) systemic simplifications. Age norms for
the occurrence of several processes will be provided, and we will then be
able to determine if Adam's speech is disordered or developing within
normal limits.

Structural Simplifications

Structural simplifications involve some alteration to the structure of a
particular word. Specifically, it is the structure of the syllables that make up
the word that is affected. Structural simplifications are sometimes known as
syllable structure processes. There are four main structural simplifications:
(1) deletion, (2) cluster reduction, (3) metathesis, and (4) epenthesis.

Deletion

A simple way to alter the structure of a word is to omit particular speech
units. Two main speech units are typically deleted: (1) consonants, and
(2) weak syllables.

Consonant Deletion

Consonant deletion is a normal phonological process for children
between the ages of 2;00 and 3;06 years. With this process, children may
omit sounds at the beginning of words. This is referred to as *initial
consonant deletion*, for example:

cat	/kæt/	→	[æt]
hit	/hɪt/	→	[ɪt]
boat	/bəʊt/	→	[əʊt]

In addition, a child may leave off consonants that appear at the ends of words. This is known as *final consonant deletion*, for example:

top	/tɒp/	→	[tɒ]
bed	/bɛd/	→	[bɛ]
man	/mæn/	→	[mæ]

Weak Syllable Deletion

In children between the ages of 2;00 and 4;00 years, whole syllables may also be deleted. The deleted syllables are characteristically unstressed. Recall that, in these so-called weak syllables, the neutral vowel frequently substitutes for the nuclear vowel. The most commonly deleted weak syllables are those that appear immediately before the stressed syllable. These are called pre-tonic syllables. Examples include:

banana	/bəˈnɑnə/	→	[ˈnɑnə]
potato	/pəˈteɪˌtəʊ/	→	[ˈteɪˌtəʊ]
pyjamas	/pəˈdʒɑməz/	→	[ˈdʒɑməz]

In addition, unstressed syllables that occur in any position after the stressed syllable may also be deleted. For example:

caravan	/ˈkærəˌvæn/	→	[ˈkæˌvæn]
octopus	/ˈɒktəˌpʊs/	→	[ˈɒkˌpʊs]
nursery	/ˈnɜsəˌrɪ/	→	[ˈnɜˌɹɪ]

Cluster Reduction

Recall that the most structurally simple words in English consist of just one vowel, eg, *a* in <u>a</u> *ball* and *I* as in <u>I</u> *know you*. Consonants can either precede a vowel to make a CV word, eg, *car* /kɑ/ and *go* /gəʊ/, or follow it to produce a VC word, eg, *ark* /ɑk/ and *oat* /əʊt/. Various combinations of consonants and vowels may occur, but most words have at least one vowel. Some words are structured with clusters of more than one consonant in a sequence. Examples include: *plan* /plæn/ (CCVC), *flow*

/fləʊ/ (CCV), *brown* /braʊn/ (CCVC), *splash* /splæʃ/ (CCCVC these examples includes a cluster at the beginning of the word. clusters involve a complicated coordination of the vocal apparatus in order to produce a smooth transition from one consonant to another, it may be too difficult for some children, depending upon their age (and, therefore, their neurological development). As a consequence, a child may delete the cluster completely, for example:

glow (CCV)   /gləʊ/   →   [əʊ]

Alternatively the cluster may be reduced by articulating only one of the consonants in the cluster, for example:

snake (CCVC)   /sneɪk/   →   [neɪk] or [seɪk]

This type of structural simplification is known as *initial cluster reduction*. Further examples include:

flower (CCV)   /flaʊə/   →   [aʊə], [faʊə] or [laʊə]
cream (CCVC)   /krim/   →   [im], [kim] or [rim]
stream (CCCVC)   /strim/   →   [im], [stim], [tim], [sim] and so on

We have noted that consonant clusters do not appear just at the beginnings of words; they can also occur at the ends of words, eg, *last* /last/ (CVCC), *halt* /hɒlt/ (CVCC), *tents* /tɛnts/ (CVCCC). As with clusters in initial position, these clusters may also be completely deleted or reduced. Examples of *final cluster reduction* include the following:

mast (CVCC)   /mast/   →   [ma], [mas] or [mat]
halts (CVCCC)   /hɒlts/ →   [hɒ], [hɒl], [hɒlt], [hɒt] and so on
mould (CVCC)   /məʊld/ →   [məʊ], [məʊl] or [məʊd]

Cluster reduction is common in children between 2;00 and 3;06 years of age.

Metathesis

This structural process involves a reordering of the sequence of consonants and vowels within a syllable. For example, in a CVC sequence the first and last consonants may be reversed, ie:

$$C_1VC_2 \quad \rightarrow \quad C_2VC_1$$

An example of this type of reordering would be when the word *teapot* /tipɒt/ is realised as [titɒp]. Here the initial C_1VC_2 sequence /pɒt/ is reversed to produce the C_2VC_1 sequence [tɒp]. Further examples include the following:

cup	/kʌp/	→	[pʌk]
football	/fʊtbɔl/	→	[tʊfbɔl]
remember	/rəmɛmbə/	→	[məɹɛmbə]

A second type of metathesis involves the resequencing of a cluster-vowel combination to produce a CVC syllable, ie:

$$C_1C_2V \rightarrow C_1VC_2$$

An example of this type of metathesis would be the word *fly* /flaɪ/ being realised as [faɪl], where the second consonant of the cluster is placed after the nuclear vowel. Further examples include:

stew	/stu/	→	[sut]
blow	/bləʊ/	→	[bəʊl]
play	/pleɪ/	→	[peɪl]

A third type of metathesis involves the reversal of the consonants within clusters that typically appear in word-final position, ie:

$$C_1C_2 \rightarrow C_2C_1$$

An example of this would be the word *mask* /mɑsk/ being realised as [mɑks]. Here, the sound elements of the cluster /-sk/ at the end of the word are reversed. Further examples include:

best	/bɛst/	→	[bɛts]
tops	/tɒps/	→	[tɒsp]
desk	/dɛsk/	→	[dɛks]

Epenthesis
Epenthesis involves the insertion of a vowel within a consonant cluster, ie:

$$CC \rightarrow CVC$$

It is usually initial consonant clusters that are affected, and typically it is the so-called 'schwa' vowel /ə/ that is inserted. An example of this would be the word *flow* /fləʊ/ being realised as [fələʊ] where the schwa is inserted between the two consonants that form the initial /fl-/ cluster of the word. Once inserted, the vowel is referred to as the epenthetic vowel. Further examples include the following:

play	/pleɪ/	→	[pələɪ]
brick	/brɪk/	→	[bəɹɪk]
snow	/snəʊ/	→	[sənəʊ]

Systemic Simplifications

Unlike the structural simplifications described, systemic simplifications do not alter the syllable structure of a word. Rather, they systematically vary a particular type of speech sound and replace it with another speech sound. Systemic simplifying processes may be divided into three types: (1) substitutions, (2) assimilations, and (3) feature synthesis. We will discuss each of these in turn.

Substitutions

There are many different types of substitutions that can be made in normally-developing speech. We will consider six of these in this subsection: (1) fronting, (2) backing, (3) stopping, (4) frication, (5) gliding, and (6) denasalisation.

Fronting

When a speech sound that is made relatively further back in the mouth is systematically substituted with a sound that is made further forwards in the mouth, it is referred to as fronting. Although in principle, this can apply to any 'back' sound, there are actually two main speech sounds that are fronted in normally-developing speech. These are the velar and palato-alveolar sounds. Recall that velar sounds are produced at the back of the mouth by the back of the tongue contacting the soft palate. Recall also that velar sounds develop after sounds made at the front of the mouth, such as bilabials and alveolars. Because of this, depending on a child's maturity, it may produce a relatively easier front sound when the adult form of the word requires that a back velar sound should be produced. In order to illustrate this, consider the word *cup* /kʌp/. This word begins with the voiceless velar plosive /k/, followed by the vowel /ʌ/, and finally by the voiceless bilabial plosive /p/. If the child finds the initial /k/ too difficult it may produce a sound at the front of the mouth such as /p/ to make [pʌp], or /t/ to make [tʌp]. In that case, the child has fronted the velar consonant and has demonstrated *syllable-initial velar fronting*. A further point to note is that when a child fronts a difficult velar consonant, the new 'front' consonant which is substituted typically has the same voicing as the velar consonant it replaces. So, if /k/, which is a voiceless consonant, is fronted the new 'front' consonant is also typically voiceless – usually /p/ or /t/. Similarly, if /g/, which is the voiced velar plosive, is fronted then the substituting consonant is also typically voiced – usually /b/ or /d/. While /p/, /b/, /t/ and /d/ are the most common sounds that are substituted for velar sounds, in theory any sound made further forward in the mouth than a velar is considered to be an example of fronting. Thus, if a child said [vəʊ] for *go* rather than the adult form /gəʊ/, as the /v/ is made further forward in the mouth than the /g/ for which it substitutes this may also be considered an example of syllable-initial velar fronting. Further examples include the following:

cat	/kæt/	→	[tæt]
goat	/gəʊt/	→	[dəʊt]
cod	/kɒd/	→	[pɒd]

The child may also front velar consonants that appear in syllable-final position; this is known as *syllable-final velar fronting*, for example:

big	/bɪg/	→	[bɪb]
hug	/hʌg/	→	[hʌd]
back	/bæk/	→	[bæt]

Finally, it is apparent that as well as the voicing typically remaining the same as the substituted velar consonant, the manner of the new consonant is also frequently consistent with that of the substituted velar consonant. So, for example, the plosives /k/ and /g/ are typically substituted by a plosive sound made further forwards in the mouth, such as /p/, /t/, /b/ or /d/, and the nasal /ŋ/ by a front nasal sound such as /m/ or /n/, for example:

wick	/wɪk/	→	[wɪp] or [wɪt]
wig	/wɪg/	→	[wɪb] or [wɪd]
wing	/wɪŋ/	→	[wɪm] or [wɪn]

Velar fronting is customary in normally-developing children between the ages of 2;00 and 3;00 years. Armed with this information, we are now able to determine whether or not the example of fronting in Adam's speech (presented earlier under the sub-heading of *Speech Disorder*) demonstrates that he has a speech disorder. Recall that Adam is 4;00 years old. This is, therefore, 1;00 year older than the expected upper age limit for the occurrence of this phonological process. In other words, we would not expect a child of 4;00 years to be continuing to front velar consonants. We would conclude, therefore, that Adam has a phonological difficulty.

We indicated earlier that, as well as velar consonants being fronted, the palato-alveolar consonants /ʃ/, /ʒ/, /tʃ/ and /dʒ/ may also be fronted. This type of fronting is referred to as *palato-alveolar fronting* and, like velar fronting, it can occur in syllable-initial or syllable-final position. Consider the word *jam* /dʒæm/ being realised as [væm]. Here, the voiced palato-alveolar affricate /dʒ/ has been substituted by a sound made further forwards in the mouth, the voiced labio-dental fricative /v/. As with velar fronting, the substituting sound usually mirrors the same voicing as the substituted palato-alveolar sound. In addition, the substituting sound typically retains the friction of the palato-alveolar fricatives and affricates. Consequently, they are commonly substituted by fricatives made further forwards in the mouth. Further examples of palato-alveolar fronting include the following:

shop	/ʃɒp/	→	[θɒp]
chair	/tʃɛə/	→	[sɛə]
jaw	/dʒɔ/	→	[ðɔ]

We know that the voiced palato-alveolar fricative /ʒ/ never occurs at the beginning of words in English. However, as with the other palato-alveolar sounds, it can be substituted in syllable-final position, for example:

garage	/gærɑʒ/	→	[gæɹɑz]
match	/mætʃ/	→	[mæs]
badge	/bædʒ/	→	[bæz]

Palato-alveolar fronting is widespread in children from the age of 2;00 years up to as old as 4;06 years.

Backing

Conceptually, backing is the reverse of fronting. While children may demonstrate idiosyncratic simplifying processes, in reality it is the alveolar plosives /t/ and /d/ that are typically 'backed'. However, the principle is, once more, that any sound made further back in the mouth than the expected target sound is considered to be an example of backing. Examples of *syllable-initial backing* include:

bun	/bʌn/	→	[gʌn]
tie	/taɪ/	→	[kaɪ]
door	/dɔ/	→	[gɔ]

In the first example, the voiced bilabial plosive /b/, which is made at the front of the mouth, is substituted by the voiced velar plosive /g/, which is made at the back of the mouth: hence the sound is said to be backed. The second example demonstrates the backing of the voiceless alveolar plosive /t/ by the substitution of the voiceless velar plosive /k/. The final example shows the front sound /d/ being backed through the substitution again of /g/. Examples of *syllable-final backing* can also be found:

put	/pʊt/	→	[pʊk]
head	/hɛd/	→	[hɛg]
tap	/tæp/	→	[tæk]

Backing is frequently observed as a normal process in children from 2;00 and 3;00 years of age.

Stopping

Recall that one of the distinguishing features of speech sounds is the manner of their articulation, ie, the type of contact made between the two articulators. We have recognised five manners of articulation: plosive, nasal, fricative, affricate and approximant. We have also noted that some speech sounds can be sustained for several seconds, while some cannot. Of the five manners of articulation described, only the plosives cannot be sustained. The remainder can all be produced and sustained for several seconds, provided there is sufficient breath support. We have learnt that plosives are generally the first speech sounds to develop and it is not until about 2;06–3;00 years of age that non-plosive sounds begin to be differentiated consistently. Thus, a further way of simplifying the production of certain words is to make sustainable sounds – especially fricatives and affricates – plosive, ie, to stop them. Recall that plosives are sometimes referred to as stops because there is a complete stopping of the airflow prior to it being released forcefully through the mouth. The process of substituting a plosive sound for a sustainable sound is therefore known as stopping. As with all the systemic simplifications discussed so far, stopping can occur in syllable-initial or syllable-final position. Consider the word *sock* /sɒk/ realised as [tɒk]. Here the sustainable voiceless alveolar fricative /s/ is stopped and replaced by the voiceless alveolar plosive /t/. Further examples of *syllable-initial stopping* include the following:

van	/væn/	→	[bæn]
sun	/sʌn/	→	[tʌn]
shop	/ʃɒp/	→	[kɒp]

The first example illustrates how the voiced labio-dental fricative /v/ is stopped by the substitution of the voiced bilabial plosive /b/. In the second example, the fricative /s/ is stopped through substitution of the plosive /t/. Finally, the syllable-initial palato-alveolar fricative /ʃ/ is stopped with the production of the velar plosive /k/. Examples of *syllable-final stopping* include:

fish	/fɪʃ/	→	[fɪt]
hiss	/hɪs/	→	[hɪt]
hose	/həʊz/	→	[həʊd]

There is a lot of variation in the chronology of stopping. Stopping of /f/ is prevalent in children between 2;00 and 2;06 years. Stopping of its voiced counterpart /v/ occurs until 3;06 years. Stopping of /s/ is common up to age 3;00 years, and its voiced partner /z/ until about 3;06 years. Stopping of /ʃ/, /tʃ/ and /dʒ/ may continue right up until the age of 4;06 years.

Frication
Frication is the name given to the process in which either a glide or a liquid (ie, an approximant) is substituted by a fricative. Consider the following examples:

yacht	/jɒt/	→	[zɒt]
yawn	/jɔn/	→	[zɔn]
we	/wi/	→	[vi]

In the first two examples the syllable-initial glide /j/ is substituted by the voiced alveolar fricative /z/. In the third example, the glide /w/ is substituted by the voiced labio-dental fricative /v/. In these examples the substituted sounds mirror the voicing of the glides, ie, they are voiced. Similar examples of substitutions for liquids can be found:

look	/lʊk/	→	[zʊk]
red	/rɛd/	→	[ðɛd]
barrow	/bærəʊ/	→	[bæðəʊ]

In the first example, the liquid /l/ is again substituted by the fricative /z/. The liquid /r/ appears in both the second and third examples. In the second example it appears in syllable-initial position and in word-initial position. In the third example it again appears in syllable-initial position but, this time, in the middle of the word. It is substituted in both cases by the voiced dental fricative /ð/, once more mirroring the voicing of the glide.

Gliding
Recall that the first two approximants to develop in a child's speech are the glides /w/ and /j/. Both consonants are usually established by the time the child reaches 3;06 years. However, the later developing liquids, /l/ and /r/ may not be fully consolidated until 6;00 years of age. The phonological simplifying process of gliding occurs when the child substitutes a glide for

a target liquid. For example, the lateral approximant /l/ in the word *yellow* /jɛləʊ/ may be substituted by the glide /w/ to give [jɛwəʊ]. Further examples of gliding include the following:

red	/rɛd/	→	[wɛd]
lolly	/lɒlɪ/	→	[jɒjɪ]
leaf	/lif/	→	[wif]

Denasalisation
This process takes place when a nasal is substituted by a homorganic plosive. Consider the following example:

| *me* | /mi/ | → | [bi] |

Here, the voiced bilabial nasal /m/ is substituted by the voiced bilabial plosive /b/. Recall that the substituting /b/ consonant is said to be homorganic because it has the same place of articulation as the /m/ consonant for which it is substituting. In this instance the voicing of the substituting sound also reflects the voicing of the sound for which it is substituting, ie, they are both voiced. As it is the nasal manner of articulation that is altered this explains why this process is referred to as denasalisation. Further examples include the following:

bun	/bʌn/	→	[bʌd]
hang	/hæŋ/	→	[hæg]
mat	/mæt/	→	[bæt]

Assimilations
Assimilation is said to have taken place when one speech segment is transposed into another owing to the influence of a neighbouring segment. In the majority of cases the segments are individual speech sounds, but there are instances where a whole syllable will influence a neighbouring syllable. As with substitutions, several assimilations are identifiable. In this subsection we will describe five of these: (1) reduplication, (2) vowel harmony, (3) consonant harmony, (4) context-sensitive voicing, and (5) word-final de-voicing.

Reduplication

Consider the following example:

    bottle   /bɒtəl/   →   [bɒbɒ]

Here, the second syllable is transposed owing to the influence of the neighbouring first syllable. In fact, it is transposed into the first syllable. In effect, the first syllable /bɒ/ is reduplicated: hence the name of this process. Assimilatory processes may be defined according to whether or not the affected segment of a word follows or precedes the segment that causes the assimilation. If the affected segment follows the segment that causes the assimilation then this is said to be progressive assimilation. In the above example, we see that the affected syllable /təl/ follows the syllable that causes the assimilation /bɒ/. Consequently, this is an example of progressive assimilation. The process of reduplication may be summarised as follows:

    syllable$_1$ syllable$_2$ →   syllable$_1$ syllable$_1$

Further examples of reduplication include the following:

    mummy   /mʌmɪ/   →   [mʌmʌ]
    David   /deɪvɪd/ →   [deɪdeɪ]
    biscuit   /bɪskɪt/ →   [bɪbɪ]

As well as reduplication being described as a progressive process, it is also a contiguous process. This means that the segment causing the assimilation is next to the affected segment. This is clearly the case in reduplication, in which the second syllable is always next to the first syllable.

Vowel harmony

This assimilatory process affects unstressed vowels such that the unstressed vowel assimilates to the vowel within the syllable that receives the primary stress. For example:

    water   /ˈwɔtə/   →   [wɔtɔ]

In this example the vowel within the unstressed second syllable is /ə/. This vowel harmonises with the /ɔ/ vowel within the syllable that receives the primary stress. In addition, this particular example is also progressive, ie, the affected segment follows the segment causing the assimilation. Further examples include the following:

meter	/ˈmitə/	→	[miti]
dinner	/ˈdɪnə/	→	[dɪnɪ]
father	/ˈfaðə/	→	[faða]

Vowel harmony need not always be progressive, however. In some instances the affected segment precedes the segment that causes the assimilation. In such cases this is known as regressive assimilation. An example of regressive vowel harmony is given below:

annoy	/əˈnɒɪ/	→	[ɒɪnɒɪ]

Here we see that the unstressed vowel /ə/ precedes the vowel /ɒɪ/ that causes the assimilation. Further examples include:

aloud	/əˈlaʊd/	→	[aʊlaʊd]
agree	/əˈgri/	→	[igri]
potato	/pəˈteɪˌtəʊ/	→	[peɪteɪtəʊ]

Unlike reduplication which is contiguous, vowel harmony is a non-contiguous process, ie, the segment that causes the assimilation is not next to the affected element: in all the examples, it can be seen that the vowels are separated from one another by consonant sounds.

Consonant Harmony
Conceptually, consonant harmony represents the counterpart process to vowel harmony: of course, with this process it is the consonants that are affected. As with vowel harmony, consonant harmony is also a non-contiguous process, the consonants being separated from each other by vowels. Consonant harmony can also be both progressive and regressive. Alveolar sounds are particularly susceptible to consonant harmony. Consider the following example:

pet	/pɛt/	→	[pɛp]

Here, the affected segment is the final /t/ which follows the segment that causes it to assimilate, ie, the initial /p/. Therefore, this is an example of progressive consonant harmony. An example of regressive consonant harmony affecting an alveolar sound is given below:

dome　　　/dəʊm/　→　[məʊm]

This time, the affected segment /d/ precedes the /m/ segment that causes the assimilation. As well as alveolar consonants harmonising to bilabial consonants they may also harmonise to velar consonants, for example:

progressive:　*gun*　　/gʌn/　→　[gʌŋ]
regressive:　*knock*　/nɒk/　→　[ŋɒk]

In both of these examples, the alveolar nasal /n/ has harmonised to the affecting velar consonant. In both cases the newly assimilated segment has retained its nasal manner of articulation, hence the production of the velar nasal [ŋ].

Context-Sensitive Voicing
Children between the ages of 2;00 and 3;00 years seem to find it easier to produce voiced consonants when they appear before a vowel, ie, in prevocalic position. The reason for this is thought to be because the voicing of the consonant 'anticipates' the immediately following voicing of the vowel. The child appears more able to commence and sustain the vibration of the vocal folds for the consonant when this is carried through into the immediately succeeding vowel. Consequently, it is easier for a child to say /bi/ than /pi/ because both the /b/ and /i/ are voiced in /bi/, but there is a variation from voiceless /p/ to voiced /i/ in /pi/. In summary, children up to the age of about 3;00 years are likely to voice systematically any voiceless consonants that precede vowels. Consider the following examples:

tea　　/ti/　　→　[di]
thin　　/θɪn/　→　[ðɪn]
sun　　/sʌn/　→　[zʌn]

In the first example, it can be seen that the voiceless alveolar plosive /t/ occurs immediately before a vowel. As it is easier for the child to produce a voiced consonant in this prevocalic context, the child substitutes the counterpart voiced alveolar plosive /d/. Similarly in the second example, the prevocalic voiceless dental fricative /θ/ is substituted with the counterpart voiced dental fricative /ð/. The final example shows the substitution of voiceless prevocalic /s/ with voiced /z/.

Word-Final De-Voicing

We have noted above that children between the ages of 2;00 and 3;00 years find it easier to produce a voiced consonant before a vowel. In contrast, children of the same age seem to find the production of voiceless consonants simpler than the production of voiced consonants when they occur at the ends of words. The reason here is thought to be that, this time, the word-final consonant 'anticipates' the upcoming silence at the end of the word. Accordingly, the child finds it easier to say /kæp/ than /kæb/. This feature may be used systematically throughout a child's speech, ie, the word-final consonant is de-voiced. We have already touched on the concept of de-voicing in the previous chapter when we considered how some phonemes are de-voiced to form new allophones, eg, [b̥] and [ɹ̥]. With word-final de-voicing, for example, the word *dab* /dæb/ may be realised as [dæb̥]. Here, the fully voiced bilabial plosive /b/, which occurs in a word-final post-vocalic position, is de-voiced and realised as [b̥]. Alternatively, and more commonly, the fully voiced plosive /b/ may lose all of its voicing, in which case it would be realised as the fully voiceless plosive [p], ie, *dab* /dæb/ → [dæp]. Further examples of word-final de-voicing include the following:

bed	/bɛd/	→	[bɛt]
nose	/nəʊz/	→	[nəʊs]
bag	/bæg/	→	[bæk]

Feature Synthesis

Clusters are often simplified by the process of feature synthesis. This occurs when the phonetic characteristics of one segment of the cluster are combined with the phonetic characteristics of the other segment, thereby yielding just one new single segment. Consider the following:

smoke	/sməʊk/	→	[m̥əʊk]

In this example, the voicelessness of the initial /s/ is combined with the bilabiality and nasality of the /m/ to produce the single voiceless bilabial nasal [m̥], ie:

voiceless /s/ + bilabial nasal /m/ = voiceless bilabial nasal [m̥]

A further example is this:

swing   /swɪŋ/   →   [ɸɪŋ]

Here, the voicelessness and frication of the initial /s/ is combined with the bilabial place of articulation of the /w/ to yield the single voiceless bilabial fricative [ɸ]. (This sound is rather like the noise made when blowing a kiss: the lips are rounded and protruded, and one then blows gently through the pursed lips.) In other words:

voiceless fricative /s/ + bilabial /w/ = voiceless bilabial fricative [ɸ]

There are many other examples of feature synthesis, but the defining characteristic is the combination of the phonetic features of one segment with those of another to yield a single segment.

Co-Occurrence of Phonological Processes

The phonological simplifying processes described in this chapter should serve to illustrate that most of the 'mistakes' children make are not really errors at all. In fact, the majority of children are still using some phonological simplifying processes up to the age of 5;00 years, and some even beyond this. As with most processes of human communication, phonological simplifying processes do not always operate in isolation from other processes, or from different presentations of the same process. For example, the process of stopping does not have to operate exclusively in either syllable-initial or syllable-final position: it may operate in both positions at the same time. This would mean that all fricatives would be stopped. So, if this were the case, the earlier example of *fish* may result in the child producing [tɪt], where the initial fricative /f/ is stopped as well as the final fricative /ʃ/. Other examples of stopping both syllable-initial and syllable-final fricatives include the following:

shoes	/ʃuz/	→	[tud]
sauce	/sɔs/	→	[tɔt]
vase	/vɑz/	→	[bɑd]

It is also common to have several processes affecting communication at any one time. Consider the following words which provide examples of two or more co-occurring processes:

stack	/stæk/	→ [tæt]	initial cluster reduction /st-/ → [t]
			fronting of syllable-final /k/ → [t]
splash	/splæʃ/	→ [æp]	deletion of initial cluster /spl-/
			stopping of syllable-final /ʃ/ → [p]
treat	/trit/	→ [tik]	initial cluster reduction /tr-/ → [t]
			backing of syllable-final /t/ → [k]
sparks	/spɑks/	→ [kɑ]	initial cluster reduction /sp-/ → [p]
			backing of the resultant /p/ → [k]
			deletion of the final cluster /-ks/
spoons	/spunz/	→ [fun]	feature synthesis /sp/ → [f]
			reduction of final cluster /-nz/ → [n]

We have now completed our discussion of English phonology operating at the syllabic and word level. The next chapter considers how the pronunciation of words may alter when they are strung together in so-called connected speech.

Revision Exercises

7.1 Name the three levels at which the speech sound system is organised.

7.2 Analyse the realisations of the following words and identify which structural phonological simplifying process (deletion, cluster reduction, metathesis, epenthesis) may be operating, eg, *dog* /dɒg/ → [dɒ] – final consonant deletion, *lamp* /læmp/ → [læm] – final cluster reduction, *rabbit* /ræbɪt/ → [bærɪt] – metathesis, *film* /fɪlm/ → [fɪləm] – epenthesis:

flag	/flæg/	→	[fæg]
snake	/sneɪk/	→	[səneɪk]
police	/pəˈlis/	→	[ˈlis]
posts	/pəʊsts/	→	[pəʊs]
case	/keɪs/	→	[seɪk]
cup	/kʌp/	→	[ʌp]
pat	/pæt/	→	[pæ]
flow	/fləʊ/	→	[fəʊl]
bring	/brɪŋ/	→	[bərɪŋ]
boat	/bəʊt/	→	[bəʊ]

7.3 Analyse the realisations of the following words and identify which systemic substitutions (fronting, backing, stopping, frication, gliding, denasalisation) may be operating, eg, *bag* /bæg/ → [bæd] – syllable-final velar fronting, *rope* /rəʊp/ → [zəʊp] – frication:

miss	/mɪs/	→	[mɪt]
look	/lʊk/	→	[zʊk]
shed	/ʃɛd/	→	[fɛd]
door	/dɔ/	→	[gɔ]
love	/lʌv/	→	[jʌv]
man	/mæn/	→	[bæn]
pig	/pɪg/	→	[pɪd]
soap	/səʊp/	→	[təʊp]
cart	/kɑt/	→	[tɑt]
badge	/bædʒ/	→	[bæz]
read	/rid/	→	[jid]
hat	/hæt/	→	[hæk]
ring	/rɪŋ/	→	[rɪg]

Activities

7.4 Make an audio recording of an informal conversation between two people. Select one of the participants as the subject and transcribe the first 300 words used by them. Determine the number of syllables in each word and then calculate the average word length in syllables for all 300 words. Also make a note of the longest and shortest words (in syllables). Next select two written articles, one from the tabloid press and one from the broadsheets. Similarly, determine the number of syllables in each of the first 300 words of both articles, together with the average word lengths. Again make a note of the longest and shortest words (in syllables) for each article. Describe your findings and explain any differences.

7.5 Make an audio recording of the speech of a 3;00-year-old child. Transcribe at least 50 words using the IPA symbols set out in Tables 6.1, 6.2 and 6.8. Identify examples of systemic substitutions. Identify any homophones that are used/created by substituting processes. How does the occurrence of these processes affect the child's intelligibility?

Note

1 *We have adopted the practice of showing how a person actually realises, or pronounces, particular sounds, syllables and words by enclosing them in square brackets [ ]. Note also that, for the sake of clarity, we do not necessarily represent all phonetic features of these realisations. We show only those features that contribute to an understanding of the argument.*

....

CHAPTER 8

Connected Speech
....

I N THE TWO PRECEDING CHAPTERS we saw how systematic operations can alter the pronunciation of words. Some of these systematic operations are due to word-internal factors, such as the allophonic variations that arise owing to the context in which speech sounds occur. For example, we have seen that the allophone [p] only occurs after a /s/ in English, and that the aspirated allophone [pʰ] occurs in all other contexts. We have also seen how certain phonological simplifying processes may alter the eventual pronunciation of words through either structural simplifications, such as deletion, or systemic simplifications, such as fronting. As well as word-internal factors, we have also noted a few operations that alter the pronunciation of a word owing to the anticipation of an upcoming silence at the end of a word, such as word-final de-voicing. All of the operations described so far operate at the syllabic and word level. However, it is self-evident that we do not normally speak using words in isolation. Rather, we string together a series of words in a verbal stream that we call connected speech. This chapter examines connected speech. First, we consider articulatory dynamics and the factors that influence the movement of the articulators when producing a stream of words in real time. We then examine how the pronunciation of words alters from their citation form when they are combined into connected speech. Specifically, four processes that influence these pronunciation changes are considered: assimilation, vowel reduction, liaison and elision. Next, we introduce the concept of prosody and discuss the role of rhythm, stress and intonation in signalling meaning in connected speech. Finally, we examine the notion of fluency and note that all connected speech contains so-called normal dysfluencies, such as repetitions, prolongations and hesitations.

Articulatory Dynamics

We have previously noted that connected speech involves rapid, coordinated, sequential movements of the articulatory mechanism. Our ability to move the articulators with precision in connected speech is influenced by two main factors: (1) the biomechanical performance of the articulatory mechanism, and (2) the neuromuscular control mechanism. Each of these factors is described below.

Biomechanical Performance

There are limits to the speed at which the articulators can move. The tongue and lips, for example, can only move so fast, the rate being influenced by their mass and size. Any massive object has a property known as inertia. That is to say, a massive object resists being set in motion. Similarly, the articulators resist being set in motion, and consequently there is a delay between the nerve impulse that initiates a movement and the performance of a particular articulatory manoeuvre. We have already considered one example of the effect of delay when we examined the process of nasalisation in Chapter 6. Recall that the vowel /ɑ/ in the word *mart* /mɑt/ is nasalised, ie, [mã̃tʰ]. The explanation for this is delay in articulatory movement. The nasality of the initial /m/ overlaps on to the following vowel, owing to a delay in raising the velum after the /m/ is articulated. Similarly, the diphthong /aʊ/ is nasalised in the word *now* /naʊ/, owing again to an inherent delay in raising the velum after the initial /n/ is articulated, ie, /naʊ/ → [naʊ̃]. The examples provided here relate to words in isolation but, as you might imagine, the effects of biomechanical performance are compounded in connected speech, where a whole series of movements must be initiated. Each time an articulator is set in motion there is always the initial inertia to be overcome.

Neuromuscular Control

The effect of the neuromuscular control system is the opposite of the articulatory delay that is induced by the biomechanical features of the articulatory mechanism. It appears that, in order to compensate for the intrinsic delays in initiating articulatory movements, the neuromuscular commands that control them may be initiated in advance of their being required. The articulatory characteristics of the target articulation may then appear on an earlier segment of speech. Once more, we were introduced to this concept when we considered allophonic nasalisation within a word. We have already reviewed how the nasalisation of vowels that follow nasal consonants may be explained by articulatory inertia. Recall also that vowels that precede a nasal consonant may be nasalised. For example, the vowel /æ/ in the name *Anne* /æn/ may be nasalised, ie, [æ̃n]. The explanation for this lies in a consideration of the neuromuscular control mechanism. In anticipation of the upcoming nasal /n/, which requires a lowered velum, the neuromuscular command to lower the velum is initiated in advance of it being required. Consequently, the articulatory characteristic of the nasality of /n/ appears on the earlier /æ/ segment, thereby nasalising the vowel. A similar argument may be applied to the word *wing* /wɪŋ/, which is typically realised as [wɪ̃ŋ]. Again, anticipating the upcoming nasal /ŋ/, and in an effort to compensate for articulatory inertia, the neuromuscular command to lower the velum is initiated in advance of it being required. Consequently, the characteristic nasality of the consonant overlaps on to the immediately prior /ɪ/ vowel. Again, the examples provided in this sub-section relate to words in isolation. However, the principle of advanced initiation of articulatory movement applies in just the same way to connected speech. For example, as the final sound in one word is being completed, the neuromuscular control mechanism may already have initiated a signal in anticipation of the upcoming first sound in the immediately following word. Therefore, the effects of the neuromuscular control mechanism extend from one word to another in connected speech, in just the same way as the effects of biomechanical performance.

So we can see how features of articulation interact and overlap. Such so-called coarticulations are especially present in connected speech, where the impact of inherent delay in the biomechanical system and the

224

compensatory mechanism of early initiation of neuromuscular commands influences the pronunciation of words (Hardcastle & Hewlett, 1999). The pronunciation of connected words is particularly prone to alteration across word boundaries, ie, where one word meets another immediately following word. Consequently, the sounds that are most affected are the sounds at the ends of words and the sounds at the beginning of words. For example, the phrase *that pen* /ðæt pɛn/ sounds more like [ðæp pɛn] in connected speech. Here the word-final /t/ of the word *that* assimilates to the place of articulation of the word-initial /p/ of the immediately following word *pen*. This, and other word boundary processes, will be discussed in detail below. Specifically, four processes will be examined: (1) assimilation, (2) vowel reduction, (3) liaison, and (4) elision. Before proceeding, however, it is worth making a general point. Sounds across word boundaries may alter, but they do not necessarily have to. The speech of a person who is particularly careful over their enunciation may not be significantly affected by processes such as assimilation, vowel reduction, liaison and elision. However, it would be unusual if none of a person's connected speech were influenced. The degree to which such processes have an impact on connected speech varies from person to person.

Assimilation

Connected speech is more than a series of target articulations strung together by simple movements. In reality, we find that individual target articulations are nearly always affected by the articulation of adjacent segments. Therefore there is often a considerable overlap of articulatory activities in connected speech – a feature known as *coarticulation* (Clark & Yallop, 1995, 85). One prominent type of coarticulation is the process of assimilation. At the word level, assimilation takes place when one speech segment is transposed into another owing to the influence of a neighbouring segment within the same word. An example of this is the dentalisation of alveolars when they occur in close proximity to dental fricatives, eg, *width* /wɪdθ/ → [wɪd̪θ]. In connected speech assimilation may also take place at word boundaries. There are two types of assimilation: (1) allophonic, and (2) phonemic. Each of these is discussed in turn below.

Allophonic Assimilation

Consider the following phrase:

bad thought   /bæd θɔt/

There is a word boundary between the word *bad* and the word *thought*. The sound at the end of the word *bad* is the alveolar /d/, and the sound at the beginning of the word *thought* is the dental fricative /θ/. Just as alveolars may become dentalised within a word when they precede dental sounds, the same process of assimilation may occur across a word boundary. Consequently, the phrase may be realised as follows:

bad thought   /bæd θɔt/   →   [bæd̪ θɔt][1]

In this instance, the final /d/ of *bad* is dentalised in anticipation of the upcoming dental /θ/ that initiates the immediately following word *thought*. This is an example of allophonic assimilation in connected speech and specifically the process of dentalisation.

Dentalisation

To summarise the above argument, assimilation occurs when one sound is altered owing to the influence of a neighbouring segment, and we have seen how alveolars may be dentalised across a word boundary when followed by a dental sound, ie:

alveolar | | dental   (where '| |' indicates the word boundary)

A further example should serve to consolidate this concept:

hot thing   /hɒt θɪŋ/

In the phrase *hot thing* the word boundary occurs between the first word *hot* and the immediately following word *thing*. The first word *hot* ends with the alveolar sound /t/. Therefore this sound precedes the word boundary. The first sound following the word boundary is the dental consonant /θ/ in the word *thing*. Consequently, the alveolar sound before the word boundary is dentalised in anticipation of the upcoming dental sound that occurs immediately after the word boundary, ie:

| *hot thing* | /hɒt θɪŋ/ | → | [hɒt̪ θɪŋ] |

Further examples of dentalisation across such word boundaries include the following:

hit this	/hɪt ðɪs/	→	[hɪt̪ ðɪs]
ten things	/tɛn θɪŋz/	→	[tɛn̪ θɪŋz]
tell that	/tɛl ðæt/	→	[tɛl̪ ðæt]

We see in the above examples how all the alveolars before the word boundaries are dentalised, as they assimilate to the place of articulation of the following dental sound. As well as dentalisation, the assimilatory process of de-voicing can also occur across word boundaries.

De-voicing

De-voicing is prevalent when a voiced plosive precedes a voiceless consonant, ie:

voiced plosive | | voiceless consonant

Consider the following example:

| *lab coat* | /læb kəʊt/ |

In the phrase *lab coat* the word boundary is, of course, between the first word *lab* and the second word *coat*. The final consonant of the first word is the voiced plosive /b/, and it is this sound that immediately precedes the word boundary. The first sound after the word boundary is the initial voiceless consonant /k/ of the second word *coat*. In anticipation of this upcoming voiceless consonant the voiced plosive /b/ is de-voiced as it assimilates the voicing of this immediately following sound. Therefore the phrase is realised as follows:

| *lab coat* | /læb kəʊt/ | → | [læb̥ kəʊt] |

Further examples include the following:

Bob Smith	/bɒb smɪθ/	→	[bɒb̥ smɪθ]
big toe	/bɪg təʊ/	→	[bɪg̥ təʊ]
hard fought	/hɑd fɔt/	→	[hɑd̥ fɔt]

In each case it is the voiced plosive before the word boundary that is de-voiced, taking on the voicing of the immediately following voiceless consonant. De-voicing across word boundaries also occurs when a voiced fricative precedes a voiceless consonant, ie:

voiced fricative | | voiceless consonant

Consider the following example:

has to   /hæz tu/

In this example, it is the word-final voiced fricative /z/ of the word *has* that precedes the word boundary. The sound occurring immediately after the word boundary is the initial voiceless consonant /t/ of the following word *to*. In instances such as this, where a voiced fricative precedes a voiceless consonant across a word boundary, the preceding voiced fricative is de-voiced. Consequently, this example is likely to be realised as follows:

has to   /hæz tu/   →   [hæz̥ tu]

Further examples include the following:

phase three   /feɪz θrɪ/   →   [feɪz̥ θɹi]
live sound   /laɪv saʊnd/   →   [laɪv̥ saʊnd]
garage paint   /gæraʒ peɪnt/ →   [gæraʒ̊ peɪnt]

We see from these examples how the voiced fricative that precedes the word boundary assimilates the voicing of the immediately following voiceless consonant and, therefore, becomes de-voiced. Again, it is the sound that precedes the word boundary that is de-voiced. These are all examples of anticipatory coarticulation. This is sometimes referred to as *right-to-left coarticulation*, ie, in the sequence A | | B, sound B influences sound A. There are, however, examples of de-voicing where it is the sound that follows the word boundary that is affected. Such examples are known as *perseverative coarticulation* or *left-to-right coarticulation*, ie, in the sequence C | | D, sound C influences sound D. An example of a perseverative, left-to-right coarticulation is when a voiceless consonant precedes a liquid, ie:

voiceless consonant | | liquid

Consider the following example:

Miss Wright   /mɪs raɪt/

The sound immediately preceding the word boundary is the word-final voiceless consonant /s/ of the first word *Miss*. This is followed immediately after the word boundary by the word-initial liquid consonant /r/ of the second word *Wright*. In this instance, it is the sound before the word boundary that affects the sound following the word boundary. Consequently, it is the liquid /r/ that assimilates the voicing of the preceding voiceless consonant, becoming de-voiced, ie:

Miss Wright   /mɪs raɪt/   →   [mɪs ɹ̥aɪt]

We see that this is an example of left-to-right coarticulation, as the sound to the left of the word boundary affects the sound to the right of the word boundary. Further examples of perseverative, left-to-right de-voicing include the following:

hot love	/hɒt lʌv/	→	[hɒt l̥ʌv]
hip length	/hɪp lɛŋθ/	→	[hɪp l̥ɛŋθ]
bike race	/baɪk reɪs/	→	[baɪk ɹ̥eɪs]

In each of these examples it is the liquid sound, either /l/ or /r/, in word-initial position immediately following the word boundary, that is assimilated. In each case the liquid assumes the voicing of the preceding voiceless consonant and is de-voiced. While there are other types of allophonic assimilation across word boundaries the foregoing discussion of nasalisation and de-voicing should be sufficient to give you a feel for the operation of this process. We will now turn our attention to the second type of assimilation – phonemic assimilation.

Phonemic Assimilation

In phonemic assimilation the new speech sounds are not allophones of the original sound but, rather, they are substituting phonemes. One of the most pervasive types of phonemic assimilation is de-alveolar assimilation.

This occurs when an alveolar sound in word-final position is followed across a word boundary by a consonant in word-initial position, ie:

alveolar | | consonant

This process of assimilation is highly predictable. So, if we know which particular alveolar occupies word-final position before the word boundary, and the nature of the consonant occupying the word-initial position of the immediately following word, we can predict which phoneme will be substituted for the alveolar. We can therefore build rules that predict the nature of the assimilation that will take place. Consider the following rule:

if	/t/ ‖	/pbm/	then	/t/ → [p]

This rule is read as follows: 'If the sound in word-final position of the word preceding the word boundary is the alveolar /t/, and if the sound in word-initial position in the word immediately following the word boundary is either /p/, /b/ or /m/, then the word-final /t/ of the word preceding the word boundary will be realised as [p].' This is probably best understood with an example. Consider the following phrase:

that pony   /ðæt pəʊnɪ/

Here, the word-final sound of the word *that* preceding the word boundary is the alveolar /t/. The sound in word-initial position in the word *pony* that immediately follows the word boundary is /p/. Consequently, according to our rule, the /t/ is realised as [p], ie:

that pony   /ðæt pəʊnɪ/   →   [ðæp pəʊnɪ]

A further example should help to make this clear. Consider the following:

fat boy   /fæt bɒɪ/

In this instance, the sound in word-final position of the word preceding the word boundary is the alveolar /t/ in the word *fat*. Further, the sound in word-initial position of the word *boy* that immediately follows the word boundary is /b/. Consequently, according to our rule, the /t/ should be realised as [p], ie:

fat boy   /fæt bɒɪ/   →   [fæp bɒɪ]

Further examples of the application of this particular rule include the following:

that pail	/ðæt peɪl/	→	[ðæp peɪl]
that bale	/ðæt beɪl/	→	[ðæp beɪl]
that male	/ðæt meɪl/	→	[ðæp meɪl]

We see then how the alveolar plosive /t/ is substituted by [p] when it precedes a bilabial consonant. In summary, the voiceless alveolar plosive is substituted by a voiceless bilabial plosive. We see from this that the substituting phoneme retains both the voicing (voiceless) and manner of articulation (plosive) of the alveolar sound for which it substitutes; it is only the place of articulation that is affected, ie, it assimilates from an alveolar into a bilabial. As you might expect, a similar rule applies to the voiced alveolar plosive /d/ when it precedes a bilabial. The following rule applies:

if	/d/ ‖	/pbm/	then	/d/ → [b]

This rule is read in the same way as the previous rule, ie: 'If the sound in word-final position of the word preceding the word boundary is the alveolar /d/, and if the sound in word-initial position in the word immediately following the word boundary is either /p/, /b/ or /m/, then the word-final /d/ of the word preceding the word boundary will be realised as [b].' Consider the following example that should demonstrate this rule in action:

mad man   /mæd mæn/

In this example, the sound in word-final position of the word *mad* that precedes the word boundary is the alveolar /d/. Also, the sound in word-initial position in the word *man* that immediately follows the word boundary is /m/. Therefore, according to the rule the word-final /d/ will be realised as [b], ie:

mad man   /mæd mæn/   →   [mæb mæn]

In this instance, the voiced alveolar plosive /d/ is substituted by the voiced bilabial plosive /b/. The affected alveolar therefore retains its voicing (voiced) and manner of articulation (plosive), but the place of articulation is changed (from alveolar to bilabial). This should now make it quite clear as to why this process is known as de-alveolar assimilation, ie, because the place of articulation is altered from alveolar. Here are some further examples of the rule that we are currently considering:

good pail   /gʊd peɪl/   →   [gʊb peɪl]
good bale   /gʊd beɪl/   →   [gʊb beɪl]
good male   /gʊd meɪl/   →   [gʊb meɪl]

It should be apparent that, in each example, the alveolar /d/ is substituted this time by [b] and not [p]. To reiterate, the voicing and manner of articulation of /d/ are retained, but the place of articulation is affected, ie, the voiced alveolar plosive is substituted by a voiced bilabial plosive. A third rule similarly applies to the alveolar nasal /n/, ie:

if	/n/	/pbm/	then	/n/ → [m]

Consider the following three examples of the application of this rule:

ten pails   /tɛn peɪlz/   →   [tɛm peɪlz]
ten bales   /tɛn beɪlz/   →   [tɛm beɪlz]
ten males   /tɛn meɪlz/   →   [tɛm meɪlz]

In each of these examples, the word-final /n/ of the word preceding the word boundary is immediately followed by a bilabial plosive. Under these conditions, the /n/ retains its voicing (voiced) and manner of articulation (nasal) but, again, the place of articulation is altered. In this case it assimilates the bilabial place of articulation of the immediately following bilabial sound. Hence, the voiced alveolar nasal /n/ is substituted by a voiced bilabial nasal /m/. It is apparent that the three rules described here operate when either an alveolar plosive or alveolar nasal precedes a bilabial across a word boundary. This may be summarised as follows:

alveolar plosive or nasal | | bilabial plosive

if	/t/	/pbm/	then	/t/ → [p]
if	/d/	/pbm/	then	/d/ → [b]
if	/n/	/pbm/	then	/n/ → [m]

There are many more rules that govern de-alveolar assimilation, but these examples are sufficient for our purposes as space does not allow an exhaustive coverage. The principle, however, is that the voicing and manner of articulation of the alveolar are retained, but the place of articulation is altered. The assimilated sound is therefore no longer an alveolar, hence the term de-alveolar assimilation. One further brief example should illustrate how this principle operates. Consider the following word boundary scenario:

alveolar fricative | | post-alveolar fricative

There are just two alveolar fricatives, /s/ and /z/. The first of these is voiceless and the second is voiced. Similarly, there are just two post-alveolar fricatives, /ʃ/ and /ʒ/. These are voiceless and voiced respectively. As we know that in de-alveolar assimilation the voicing and manner of articulation of the alveolar are retained, and that only the place of articulation is altered, we would expect the voiceless alveolar fricative to be substituted by a voiceless post-alveolar fricative, and the voiced alveolar fricative to be substituted by a voiced post-alveolar fricative. In fact, this is exactly what happens. This rule may be summarised as follows:

if	/s/	/pbm/	then	/s/ → [ʃ]
if	/z/	/pbm/	then	/z/ → [ʒ]

A couple of examples should serve to demonstrate the application of this rule. Consider the following:

this shot   /ðɪs ʃɒt/

Here, the word-final consonant of the word immediately preceding the word boundary is the /s/ of the word *this*. The /s/ is a voiceless alveolar fricative. Now, the word-initial consonant in the word *shot* that follows the word boundary is the post-alveolar fricative /ʃ/. According to our rule, under these circumstances the /s/ will be substituted by a /ʃ/, ie:

this shot /ðɪs ʃɒt/ → [ðɪʃ ʃɒt]

We see that the voiceless alveolar fricative /s/ has retained its voicing (voiceless) and manner of articulation (fricative), but that it has assimilated the place of articulation of the immediately following sound (post-alveolar). Similarly, in the following example the word-final voiced alveolar fricative /z/ is substituted by the voiced post-alveolar fricative /ʒ/:

those shots /ðəʊz ʃɒts/ → [ðəʊʒ ʃɒts]

This concludes our discussion of the process of assimilation in connected speech. We will now consider each of the processes of vowel reduction, liaison and elision in turn.

Vowel Reduction

Recall that in Chapter 3 we introduced the concept of a citation form. This referred to the present tense form of a verb that is used as the main listing in dictionaries. In addition, a citation form may also be thought of as the way in which a word is pronounced when it is spoken in isolation. Thus the word *of*, in isolation, is pronounced as /ɒv/. However, in connected speech the pronunciation of this word may alter. For example:

man of means /mæn ɒv minz/ → [mæn əv minz]

Here, the so-called strong form of the word /ɒv/ is reduced to the weak form [əv]. Substituting the neutral vowel /ə/ in weak syllables is a common feature in connected speech, known as vowel reduction. Consider again the following example:

a perfect life /ə ˈpɜfɛkt ˈlaɪf/

The citation form of the indefinite article *a* is pronounced /eɪ/. However, when it appears within the above connected speech the vowel is reduced once more to the neutral schwa vowel [ə]. Now reconsider the following example:

to perfect life   /tʊ pəˈfɛkt ˈlaɪf/

We know that the citation form of the word *to* is pronounced as /tu/. However, in this example of connected speech the long vowel /u/ is reduced to the shorter vowel [ʊ]. So this is another example of vowel reduction operating in connected speech. The word *and* is another word that frequently undergoes reduction to a weak form. In isolation, it is pronounced as /ænd/, but in connected speech it may be realised as [ənd], [ən], [nd] or [n̩]. For example:

fish and chips	/fɪʃ ænd tʃɪps/	→	[fɪʃ ənd tʃɪps]
war and peace	/wɔ ænd pis/	→	[wɔ ən pis]
knife and fork	/naɪf ænd fɔk/	→	[naɪf nd fɔk]
bread and butter	/brɛd ænd bʌtə/	→	[brɛd n̩ bʌtə]

It should be noted, however, that the strong form of words may be used in connected speech. In the case of *and*, it may be used for emphasis in order to signal a contrast, as in the following:

I want bread AND butter   /aɪ wɒnt brɛd ˈænd bʌtə/

The use of the strong form in this context signals the contrast that the speaker wants both bread AND butter, and not EITHER bread OR butter.

Liaison

When a word with a vowel in word-final position is followed immediately by another word that has a vowel in word-initial position, then the two words may be linked by the insertion of an /r/ sound. Consider the following example:

more over   /mɔ əʊvə/

The first word *more* has the vowel /ɔ/ in word-final position. This is immediately followed by another word *over* that has a vowel in word-initial position, ie, the vowel /əʊ/. Under these circumstances, with one vowel following another, the two words may be linked by the insertion of an /r/ sound, ie:

more over   /mɔ əʊvə/   →   [mɔr əʊvə]

A further example should make this clear:

father of the bride /faðə əv ðə braɪd/

Consider just the first two words of this phrase, *father* and *of*. The first word *father* has the schwa vowel /ə/ in word-final position. After the word boundary, the immediately following word *of* also has the schwa vowel in word-initial position. This is because the citation form /ɒv/ has undergone vowel reduction in connected speech to [əv]. Under such circumstances, with one vowel immediately following another across a word boundary, the two words may be coupled by the insertion of the sound /r/, ie:

father of the bride /faðə əv ðə braɪd/ → [faðər əv ðə braɪd]

Here are some more examples:

lend me your ears	/lɛnd mi jɔ ɪəz/	→	[lɛnd mi jɔr ɪəz]
law and order	/lɔ ən ɔdə/	→	[lɔr ən ɔdə]
here and now	/hɪə ən naʊ/	→	[hɪər ən naʊ]

Liaison is a feature of the speech of most speakers of English. The insertion of /r/, as exemplified, is sometimes referred to by those who adhere to a prescriptive grammar, and hence a prescriptive phonology, as *intrusive 'r'*. This value-laden label again reflects an artificial notion of what constitutes 'good' speech and what constitutes 'bad' speech. For functional phonologists, it is sufficient merely to describe the processes that are commonly used by native speakers of a particular language.

Elision

Elision is the removal or deletion of a sound, or sounds. In Chapter 7 we noted elisions within words as consonant deletion, eg, *dog* /dɒg/ → [dɒ], *back* /bæk/ → [æk], and cluster reduction, eg, *flower* /flaʊə/ → [faʊə], *last* /lɑst/ → [lɑs]. Elision also occurs across word boundaries in connected speech, and it particularly affects consonant clusters. This is especially so when a word-final cluster before a word boundary is made up of a continuant sound plus a /t/, which is then followed by a word-initial consonant after the word boundary. This statement may be summarised into a rule as follows:

(continuant + /t/) | | consonant

if	/-ft/	C	then	/-ft/ → [-f]
if	/-st/	C	then	/-st/ → [-s]
if	/-ʃt/	C	then	/-ʃt/ → [-ʃ]

Consider the following phrase as an example of the application of the above rule:

laughed loudly   /lɑft lɑʊdlɪ/

We see that there is a cluster /-ft/ in word-final position in the word *laughed* before the word boundary. This is made up of the continuant sound /f/ plus /t/. This cluster is then followed by a word-initial consonant in the word *loudly* immediately after the word boundary. In instances like these, it is the /t/ that is elided, thereby reducing the consonant cluster from /-ft/ to /-f/, ie:

laughed loudly   /lɑft lɑʊdlɪ/   →   [lɑf lɑʊdlɪ]

Some further examples should make this clear:

coughed badly	/kɒft bædlɪ/	→	[kɒf bædlɪ]
best day	/bɛst deɪ/	→	[bɛs deɪ]
lashed log	/læʃt lɒg/	→	[læʃ lɒg]

In each of the above examples, there is a cluster in word-final position in the word that precedes the word boundary. Each cluster is composed of a continuant sound plus /t/, ie, /-ft/, /-st/ and /-ʃt/. Each of these sounds is then followed by a consonant in word-initial position immediately following the word boundary, ie, /b/, /d/ and /l/ respectively. In each instance the /t/ is elided, thereby reducing the cluster to just the continuant sound. As well as the occurrence of elision when the word-final cluster is composed of a continuant sound plus /t/, elision also occurs when the cluster is made up of a continuant plus /d/. There are more clusters of this nature that end in /d/ than those that end in /t/. Below we present a summary of this rule with examples:

(continuant + /d/) | | consonant

if	/-ðd/	C	then	/-ðd/ → [-ð]
if	/-vd/	C	then	/-vd/ → [-v]
if	/-nd/	C	then	/-nd/ → [-n]
if	/-zd/	C	then	/-zd/ → [-z]
if	/-ld/	C	then	/-ld/ → [-l]

bathed quickly	/beɪðd kwɪklɪ/	→	[beɪð kwɪklɪ]
shoved Billy	/ʃʌvd bɪlɪ/	→	[ʃʌv bɪlɪ]
hand towel	/hænd taʊəl/	→	[hæn taʊəl]
amused boy	/əmjuzd bɔɪ/	→	[əmjuz bɔɪ]
cold boy	/kəʊld bɔɪ/	→	[kəʊl bɔɪ]

As with assimilation, there are further rules that govern elision. We do not have space to consider these further, but the above examples should give you an idea of the principles of elision in connected speech. This completes our discussion of sounds in connected speech. We now turn our attention to prosody, and consider aspects of rhythm and intonation in conveying meaning in connected speech.

Prosody

In the previous chapter we saw how the speech sound system can be organised into various segments, ie, phonemes, syllables and words. However, there are features of connected speech that are not readily identifiable as discrete segments. Their effects go beyond single segments and affect the whole utterance. These are features such as: (1) rhythm, and (2) intonation. Such features are often referred to as *prosodic* or *suprasegmental* features. We will use the term prosodic features here, as it avoids the erroneous assumption often associated with the term suprasegmental, that these features are an afterthought, something superimposed on an utterance after its creation. Prosodic features are, in fact, an integral part of any utterance, being simultaneously compiled with the segmental features during the production of an utterance. We will consider both prosodic features in turn, beginning with rhythm.

Rhythm

We have already noted that some syllables in polysyllabic words may naturally be given more emphasis than others, ie, they are stressed. Other syllables are either given less stress or no stress at all. The occurrence of stressed and unstressed syllables in connected speech provides a characteristic beat or rhythm to the speech. Consider the following utterance:

I ˈlike to ˈeat aˈlone

This utterance appears to divide up naturally into three beats. Each beat, in this instance, is two syllables long. The first syllable of each beat is unstressed and the second syllable is stressed. Now consider the following utterance:

my ˈmother ˈlives at ˈhome

Again, this utterance appears to divide naturally into three beats. On this occasion, however, the first beat is made up of three syllables, with the primary stress on the second syllable of the beat. The second beat is made of just one syllable and this receives the primary stress. The final beat is constructed of two syllables and the primary stress rests on the second syllable. A beat is simply a unit of rhythm and it is often referred to as a *foot*. The characteristic of a foot depends upon where the primary and secondary stresses naturally occur. However, owing to the flexibility of the vocal apparatus it is possible for speakers to exploit the mechanism of stressing particular syllables in order to signal different meanings. Consider how you might stress the underlined words in the following question-answer sequence in order to make the meaning of the utterances as clear as possible:

Q: Is <u>Susan</u> Routledge today's lecturer?
A: No, <u>Margaret</u> Routledge is today's lecturer.

By stressing the word *Susan* in the question this makes it explicit to the listener that the speaker is unsure as to whether it is to be *Susan* or *Margaret Routledge* who will deliver the lecture. By stressing the word *Margaret* in the answer this makes it definite which of the sisters will be lecturing. In each instance the extra stress is likely to fall on the first syllable of the stressed word, ie:

Q: Is 'Susan Routledge today's lecturer?
A: No, 'Margaret Routledge is today's lecturer.

Stress on particular words is principally achieved by raising the pitch and increasing the volume of the syllable that receives the primary stress in the word. Let us take a few moments to consider how the vocal apparatus operates to achieve these effects.

Pitch

The pitch of the voice refers to how high or low the note produced by the vibrating vocal folds appears to be. The faster the vocal folds vibrate the higher the perceived pitch. Conversely, slowly vibrating folds will produce a lower pitch. The pitch of the note is measured by its frequency in Hertz (Hz), ie, the number of vibrations per second. The optimum pitch for the speaking voice varies from person to person but, typically, men speak with a lower pitch than women. The optimum pitch of an adult male's voice is typically within the range 120–141 Hz, and an adult female's within the range 197–227 Hz. Humans can make considerable voluntary variations to the pitch of their voices, but how is this achieved? Well, consider the sound produced by blowing across a stretched elastic band. If the elastic band is thin it has less mass and will be able to move more quickly, and the note produced is higher in pitch. If you now change this elastic band for a thicker one the note produced will be lower (provided you are blowing at the same intensity and the band is stretched the same amount). This is because the thicker elastic band has greater mass and therefore it moves more slowly. The resultant pitch is consequently perceived to be lower. Another way to alter the pitch, while blowing across the same elastic band, is to stretch it further. By increasing the tension in the elastic this has a similar effect to making the elastic band thinner. It moves more quickly and the pitch is higher. With respect to the human larynx it is not possible to change the vocal folds for a thinner set every time we wish to produce a higher pitch! Therefore, the major mechanism for altering pitch is to variously stretch and relax the vocal folds. This is achieved largely through rotational and sliding movements of the arytenoid cartilages and the tilting of the cricoid cartilage in relation to the thyroid cartilage. Human speech is usually produced in the range of about 100–10,000 Hz.

Volume

Whereas pitch is determined by the rapidity of the vibrations of the vocal folds, volume is determined by the intensity of vibration. This is controlled mainly by the force with which the air from the lungs is allowed to pass through the larynx. You will know yourself that in order to shout you need to take a large breath and expel it forcefully: it is not possible to shout loudly with a minimal amount of air. It is important to understand that the pitch of the voice can remain constant while the volume of that particular pitch can be varied. In other words, it is possible to keep the frequency of vibration the same, but to increase the strength of the vibration by forcing more air through the larynx. This means that the resultant speech sound wave produces greater motion in the air molecules. These, therefore, strike the ear drum of the listener more forcefully and the sound is perceived to be louder. Volume is measured in decibels (dB). A whispering person is typically speaking at a volume of around 10 dB. For comparison, someone shouting may be doing so at around 70–80 dB, and a jet engine will create a volume of about 110 dB. Anything above 110 dB usually creates a sensation of pain. This is known as the pain threshold for hearing.

There is actually a third method of stressing particular syllables in order to signal different meanings, and this is lengthening of the nuclear vowel. This simply means that vocalisation of the vowel is continued for a slightly longer duration than would normally be required. To summarise, we are able to stress particular words by increasing the pitch and volume of the syllable that receives primary stress and also by lengthening the nuclear vowel. This allows speakers to create differential meanings through prosodic features, for example:

1   JOHN kicked the ball
2   John KICKED the ball
3   John kicked the BALL

Utterance 1 stresses the word *John*. This stress can be seen to perform a contrastive function, ie, it differentiates the fact that it was John who kicked the ball and not some other person. Similarly, utterance 2 stresses the word *kicked*. This serves to indicate that the ball was not caught, painted, carried, etc, but that is was, in fact, kicked. Finally, utterance 3 places the stress on the word *ball*, thereby serving to make explicit what was kicked, ie, it was not a wall, grass, car, or any other object or person, it was in reality a ball. Therefore, stress on words can remove ambiguity. Consider the following celebrated example:

he fed her dog biscuits

If the stress is placed on the word *biscuits*, ie, *he fed her dog BISCUITS*, then he is feeding the dog. However, if the stress is placed on the word *dog*, ie, *he fed her DOG biscuits*, then he is feeding the woman dog biscuits!

Intonation

As well as a characteristic beat or rhythm to connected speech, as a product of stress patterns, there is also an attendant musical quality, defined by distinctive pitch changes known as tones. There are two main tones in English: (1) falling, and (2) rising. Consider the effects of both a rising and falling tone on the single-word utterance *no* (falling tone is marked with a '\' preceding the relevant syllable, and rising tone is marked with a '/' preceding the relevant syllable):

1   \ NO
2   / NO

As the word *no* is monosyllabic there is only one syllable to receive the primary stress. This is indicated by capital letters. The first utterance, with falling tone, is most likely interpretable as being a refusal, or a statement. In contrast, the second utterance, with rising tone, is probably interpretable as a questioning utterance. So we see that tone is capable of signalling meaning. In addition, we saw in Chapter 4 how longer utterances are divided into 'semantic chunks' – units of meaning that appear to convey a complete thought. These units of information are also typically marked by tonal changes – a series of rises and falls in pitch. They are known as tone groups. Each tone group has a nucleus. This is the most prominently stressed syllable in the tone group. Consider the following utterances that consist of just one tone group each:

1   he ate the \ BUN
2   he ate the / BUN

In both utterances it is the monosyllabic word *bun* that receives the prominent stress; this is, therefore, the nucleus. However, in the first utterance the nucleus receives a falling tone and in the second a rising tone. The effect of this is to alter the intended meaning. The first utterance is most likely interpretable as a matter-of-fact statement, whereas the second utterance is probably interpretable as a questioning utterance. Now consider the following extensions of these two utterances into utterances that contain two tone groups (where '|' marks the boundary between the two tone groups):

1   he ate the \ BUN | because he was \ HUNGry
2   he ate the / BUN | because he was / HUNGry

We see that these utterances divide into two units of information: (1) *he ate the bun*, and (2) *because he was hungry*. Each of these units is a tone group that contains its own nucleus. We have already identified the nucleus of the first tone group as the monosyllabic word *bun*. In the second tone group the nucleus is the first syllable of the word *hungry*. In the first utterance both tone groups receive a falling tone, and this enhances our interpretation of the utterance as a statement. Similarly, both the tone groups of the second utterance receive a rising tone, and this further accentuates our interpretation of the utterance as a question. Of course, in utterances with more than one tone group, the tones do not all have to be the same. Consider the following:

do you drink / RED | or do you drink \ WHITE

Two meaning units are identifiable in this utterance: (1) *do you drink red*, and (2) *or do you drink white*. In the first tone group the nucleus is the monosyllabic word *red*. This receives a rising tone which, as we have seen, frequently signals a question. In the second tone group the nucleus is the monosyllabic *white*. This nucleus receives a falling tone which we have, so far, identified as typically signalling a statement. The overall

243

meaning of the complete utterance, however, is interpretable as being a question, despite the fact that a falling tone is included. As well as having rising and falling tones in different tone groups it is also possible to identify two other combination tones that can occur within the same tone group. The first is a combination falling-rising tone (marked as '$\vee$'), and the second is a combination rising-falling tone (marked as '$\wedge$'). Consider the effects of these tones, again on the single-word utterance *no*:

1    $\vee$ NO
2    $\wedge$ NO

The first utterance, with its falling-rising tone, appears to be expressing disbelief. The second utterance, with its rising-falling tone, is interpretable as scolding, as when censuring a young child. In all of the examples of intonation presented so far, there have been no words following any of the nuclei of the tone groups. Of course, it is possible to have words following a nucleus. Consider the following example:

he ate the \ BUN *with ham and cheese*

In this utterance, four words *with ham and cheese* are appended after the nucleus *bun*. The words that occur after a nucleus in a tone group are known as the tail. In this instance, therefore, *with ham and cheese* represents the tail of the tone group. Now, the pitch contour of the tail always follows in the same direction as the nucleus. So, in the above example, as the nucleus receives a falling tone, then the pitch of the tail will also fall, being spread across the whole length of the tail. This may be represented diagrammatically as follows:

he ate the \ BUN with ham and cheese

This utterance continues to be interpretable as a statement. Similarly, when the nucleus in the above utterance receives a rising tone, then the pitch of the tail continues in this direction across the full length of the tail, ie:

he ate the / BUN with ham and cheese

Once more, this utterance continues to be interpretable as a question. There are several more nuances of intonation that could be investigated, but this is sufficient for our purposes as space does not permit a more detailed examination. The foregoing discussion will have demonstrated the ways in which intonation contours may be used to signal meaning. The study of intonation is clearly complex, but it is sufficient for now to recognise that people rely on intonation to clarify meanings and to interpret the attitude of the speaker. Often, the most effective communicators are perceived as those people who can effortlessly vary prosodic features to create interesting and colourful speech that is capable of expressing a diversity of intellectual and emotional meaning. In contrast, for example, a speaker who does not vary their intonation contour, according to the context of the conversation, speaks in a monotone that may be perceived as boring or disinterested. Effortlessness, however, should not be interpreted as perfection. As we will see in the next section, even the most effective communicators make several unplanned interruptions to the flow of their speech.

Fluency

We have seen how segmental features of speech are affected when words are combined into the continuous stream known as connected speech. In addition, we have noted how non-segmental features, such as rhythm and intonation, are composed simultaneously with this ongoing combination of speech segments. The aim of this planning and control is the real-time production of fluent, rhythmical speech that is readily interpretable by the listener. We have already identified two factors that influence the pronunciation of words when they are combined in real time. They are the biomechanical performance of the articulatory mechanism and the neuromuscular control of the vocal apparatus. The foregoing discussion may have given the impression that the system is fail-safe. However, this is far from accurate. Even though the neuromuscular control mechanism may initiate articulatory movements in advance of their being required, in an effort to overcome the inertia of the articulators, these signals may not always be timed precisely. As a consequence, a target articulation may not always be achieved. The signal may come a little too early, or a little too late. Consequently, the production of connected speech may not be as smooth and fluent as one might suppose. In addition to these mechanical and neurological factors, there are also linguistic planning factors to be taken into consideration. We noted in Chapter 1, when we considered the Communication Chain, that a speaker has first to decide what they wish to say, then choose the right symbols from the lexicon, then encode these into the words of the language, then select the appropriate speech sounds to represent these words before, finally, articulating the appropriate combination of words. Once more, the rapidity of communicating through connected speech makes considerable demands on the speaker's ability to plan and formulate their thoughts at the mind and linguistic level. It is expectable, therefore, that from time to time there will be hesitancies in the planning and thought processes. The speaker may also begin composing a particular word combination and then change their mind and set off in another direction. The overall effect of factors such as these is that connected speech is not 100 per cent fluent. On the contrary, during the course of a normal conversation most speakers make several unplanned repetitions of words or syllables, prolongations of sounds, and hesitations. As indicated, these features of talk tend to break up the smooth, rhythmical flow of speech and create dysfluency. Each of these features of talk is described briefly below.

Repetitions
There are four broad types of repetition exhibited in talk. These are repetitions of:

1   sounds, eg, *I w … w … w … won't*
2   syllables, eg, *it's my bo … bo … bo … bottle*
3   words, eg, *the boy has … has … has … has it*
4   phrases, eg, *I want to … I want to … I want to go*

We all make several unplanned repetitions in the course of a conversation, and this is quite normal. For children between 3;00 and 4;00 years of age about 90 per cent of the repetitions they make are repetitions of words and phrases. Less than 10 per cent of repetitions are of sounds or syllables.

Prolongations

During normal talk, certain speech sounds may be prolonged:

1   consonants, eg, *wwwwww-what is it?* and *shhhhh-show me*
2   vowels, eg, *daaaaa-ddy, muuuuu-mmy*

Prolongation of consonants is more common than prolongation of vowels. Normally, however, these prolongations last less than one second and usually occur less than once per 100 words spoken.

Hesitations

This is another fairly typical feature of normal speech. The person may be engaged in some lengthy conversation, responding to a question or whatever, and they pause for a moment before continuing with an utterance. Such hesitations can appear anywhere in an utterance, at the beginning, middle or end. There are two types of pauses:

1   silent, eg, *and I went* ... (pause for 3 seconds*)* ... *home then*
2   filled, where the silence is filled with vocalisations, such as: *erm, uh, oh*, eg, *and I went ... erm ... home then*

As we see, the above-mentioned features of talk tend to break up the smooth, rhythmical flow of speech. However, they are characteristic of everyone's connected speech. To this extent, we can say that all people are 'normally dysfluent'. The extent to which these dysfluencies pervade someone's speech, however, is dependent upon many factors. They are more likely to occur in unrehearsed, spontaneous conversation than they are in the talk of someone who has pre-prepared a speech or who is reading from a text. Psycho-social factors will also influence the occurrence of these features. For example, if the speaker is particularly nervous, or is speaking about an embarrassing topic, then it is more likely that these hesitancies will occur. Psycho-social pressures appear to influence the speaker's ability to plan their linguistic output. For the most part, however, the frequency of occurrence of repetitions, prolongations and hesitations in a person's speech does not unduly affect their ability to communicate effectively. They are seen as a natural by-product of connected speech and deemed to be within normal limits.

Blocks

For the sake of completion, it is worth noting that there is a fourth feature that may affect the fluency of connected speech. This is known as *blocking*. It occurs when two articulators come together with excessive force, eg, when the two lips come together to form the plosive sound /b/. Rather than parting the two articulators rapidly and easily, the speaker is unable to release the contact between them and a great deal of tension may build up. In severe cases a speaker may be unable to release a blocked sound for anything up to one minute. Clearly, this is a severe hindrance to the production of fluent speech. It is not, however, a feature of normal dysfluency. This feature occurs only in people whose dysfluencies are so intrusive that they are considered to be stammering, ie, the frequency of occurrence of any involuntary repetitions, prolongations, hesitations or blocks is so great that it severely disrupts their communication attempts. In addition, people who stammer often exhibit associated behaviours such as facial tics, grimacing, avoiding eye contact, covering the mouth with the hand, and sputtering, ie, an intense blast of breath following a halt in the flow of speech. Invariably, speakers are aware of the negative disruptive effects of these features on their connected speech.

This concludes our discussion of the segmental and non-segmental aspects of connected speech. In the next chapter we consider the organisation of connected speech into the social interactions that we call conversations.

Revision Exercises

8.1 Transcribe the following utterances using the IPA symbols set out in Tables 6.1, 6.2 and 6.8, taking into account any possible (phonemic) assimilations, eg, *that pan* /ðæt pæn/ → [ðæp pæn], *had been* /hæd bin/ → [hæb bin]:

this shoe	*red pen*
matt black	*bad boy*
hit me	*seven pairs*
his ship	*then make it*
Miss Shepherd	*those shells*

8.2 Make a broad transcription of the following utterances, taking into account any possible vowel reductions, liaisons or elisions, eg, *joint of lamb* /dʒɔɪnt ɒv læm/ → [dʒɔɪnt əv læm], *more on* /mɔ ɒn/ → [mɔr ɒn]:

last time	*more of it*
left bank	*mashed potato*
banned substance	*here and now*

8.3 Name two types of dysfluency that occur naturally in connected speech.

Activities

8.4 We have noted that sounds across word boundaries may alter, but they do not necessarily have to. Reflect on the way your own pronunciation is altered in connected speech. Are there some processes (assimilation, vowel reduction, liaison, elision) that are always used and some that are never used? Does one process predominate? Now consider why this may be the case. Are your pronunciations typical of others who speak with the same accent or who come from the same geographical area? Is your production influenced by what you consider to be 'correct' speech? Why do you hold the views you do? Can your production be explained by your age, gender or occupation?

8.5 Make a 10-minute audio recording of an informal conversation between two adults. Select one of the adults and identify the total number of repetitions, prolongations, hesitations and blocks in five minutes'-worth of the selected adult's speech. Work out the average number of dysfluencies per minute. Repeat this exercise using a video or audio recording of a news presenter. Similarly chart the number of each type of dysfluency in five minutes of the presenter's talk. Is there a difference in the results? Why? Did the occurrence of dysfluencies appear excessive in either case? Did the dysfluencies interfere with communication?

Note

1 *As in the previous chapter, for the sake of clarity we will not necessarily represent all phonetic features of these realisations. We will show only those features that contribute to an understanding of the argument.*

CHAPTER 9

Conversation

I N PRECEDING CHAPTERS we have seen how language is the predominant means by which humans communicate. We have noted that the symbols of language are morphemes and that these are combined on a principled basis into words, phrases and clauses. In addition, we have noted that the primary medium of language transmission is speech. The building blocks of speech have been identified as phonemes and we have seen how these too are systematically combined in order to encode the acoustic representation of words. We have also seen how the pronunciation of words may alter according to phonological rules that govern the speech sound system, and how the articulation of words is especially prone to alteration in connected speech. Moreover, we have examined non-segmental features of speech, such as rhythm and intonation, that are simultaneously compiled with the segmental features of speech sound combination in real time. All of this richness of detail underpins the creation of meaningful utterances. We have examined some aspects of the meaning of utterances when we considered semantics, and we have also touched upon the concept of the social use of language during our discussion of pragmatics. There is a sense in which all of these linguistic formulations serve a social function. As we noted in the first chapter, human communication is an intentional act performed by a human agent for the purpose of causing some effect in an attentive human recipient. By definition, therefore, this is a social act: it takes at least two people to communicate. We have already noted, and by implication rejected, the idea that communication in human societies is simply a one-way flow of information from one agent to one recipient. It is self-evident that the human compulsion to communicate finds its most powerful expression in the conduct of reciprocal conversation, the archetypal language use through which people participate in social interactions. As Schiffrin (1994, 232) points out, 'Conversation is a source of much of our sense of social order'. Linguistically, conversation also manifests its own order and this is the subject of the current chapter. As you will appreciate, there is much that could be discussed in relation to conversation, such as how it is initiated, how it is collaboratively closed down, how topics are either maintained or changed, and so on. However, we will limit ourselves here to a general consideration of how conversations are structured and how turns at talk are allocated to the participants. First, we set out some of the defining characteristics of conversation. Second, we introduce the notion of adjacency pairs as a fundamental unit of conversation. Third, we examine how turns at talk are allocated in real time and introduce a set of rules that is capable of explaining this allocation. Fourth, we examine the phenomenon of overlapping talk. We use the rules of turn allocation to explain why certain types of overlap are considered to be accidental and others to be wilful interruptions. Finally, we demonstrate two means by which conversational participants resolve the conflict of overlapping talk.

Characteristics of Conversation

Conversation is a unique human activity and there are several defining characteristics:

1   *No predetermined cognitive map*. We noted in Chapter 1 that language is stimulus-free. In support of this we considered a hypothetical situation in which a number of people were shown the painting of the *Mona Lisa*. We recognised that there would be no sure way of predicting what each person might say when presented with the portrait. They might be just as likely to say, 'What a beautiful picture', as, 'That reminds me of my sister', or any number of things. In the same way that we cannot predict that a particular stimulus will result in a particular

utterance, there is no way we can guarantee what will be said in a conversation. In other words, when two or more people converse, there is no possibility of predicting the actual utterances. Nor can we predict the size of these utterances, their order of occurrence or their relative distribution among the participants. Therefore, each conversation is a unique creative event that unfolds in real time. When we enter a conversation we have no predetermined cognitive map of how the conversation will unfold. We may have an idea of what we would like to talk about, what messages we would wish to convey, and so on, but there can be no guarantee that we will fulfil such aims.

2   *Collaboratively achieved*. Conversation requires the active participation of at least two attentive people, each performing intentional acts designed to cause some effect in the other. The current speaker strives to ensure that they are being attended to, heard and understood, while the current listener endeavours to indicate to the speaker if they have succeeded. The participants thus collaborate to construct a successful conversation.

3   *Managed on a turn-by-turn basis*. Conversation usually proceeds on an 'I say something – you say something' scheme, with one participant taking up a turn at talk immediately following the talk of the previous speaker. Thus, the roles of listener and speaker will continually alternate. At one moment I may be the speaker, with the other participant(s) acting as listener(s), but when I have finished speaking I become a current listener and another participant becomes the current speaker.

4   *One-at-a-time talk*. A general feature of conversation is that only one participant talks at any one time. This is true of most peoples in Europe and North America. However, there is some evidence to suggest that one-at-a-time talk may not be universal (Reisman, 1974). It would appear, however, that the general likelihood is that conversational participants talk one at a time.

5   *Highly coordinated.* When one speaker stops talking another takes over with very little overlap and an extremely short pause between turns. This gap between one speaker finishing their turn at talk and another participant beginning their turn at talk is so short that it has to be measured in microseconds.

To summarise, conversations are highly coordinated, collaborative events that generally have no more than one person speaking at a time, and which proceed without a predetermined cognitive map, being constructed on a turn-by-turn basis. We will now consider how conversations are broadly structured through what are known as adjacency pairs.

Adjacency Pairs

Schegloff and Sacks (1973) noted that conversations appear to be made up of sequences of two utterances. They identified four characteristics or conditions of such sequences, as follows:

1   The utterances are adjacent.
2   They are produced by different speakers.
3   They are ordered as a first part and a second part.
4   They are typed so that a particular first part requires a particular second part.

In addition, they pointed out that when the current speaker has produced a first pair part they should stop speaking and the next speaker should produce a second pair part at that juncture. These paired utterances are referred to as *adjacency pairs* and they appear to be a fundamental unit of conversation. To understand these characteristics better, consider the following simple example:

1   John   Hello   [GREETING]
2   Kath   Hi   [GREETING]

Here, the first pair part of the adjacency pair is the utterance *hello* in line 1. This type of utterance may be defined as a greeting. Therefore, the first pair part is typed (as a greeting). We have noted that a characteristic of adjacency pairs is that they are typed so that a particular first part requires a particular second part. It should be readily discernible that in general conversation greetings are usually followed by greetings. Consequently, when the first pair part is a greeting then the required second pair part is also a greeting. It is relevant, therefore, that after a greeting is uttered the current speaker should stop speaking and the next speaker should produce the relevant second pair part greeting at that juncture. Failure to produce the required second pair part greeting would be noticeable to the conversational participants. In fact, in our example, John does stop speaking and Kath produces the relevant, and required, second pair part greeting *Hi* in line 2. We see, then, in this brief extract how (1) the utterances are adjacent, (2) they are produced by different speakers, (3) they are ordered as a first part and a second part, and (4) they are typed. Now consider the following pair of utterances:

| 1 | Neil | Would you like a cup of tea? | [QUESTION] |
| 2 | Parmjit | Yes please | [ANSWER] |

In this brief sequence, Neil utters the first pair part *Would you like a cup of tea?* in line 1, which is interpretable as a question. Now, it is relevant that a question is followed by an answer. We can state, therefore, that when the first pair part of an adjacency pair is typed as a question, then the expected second pair part is typed as an answer. The person who has uttered the first pair part should then stop speaking and the next speaker should produce a second pair part at that juncture In fact, in the above extract, this is exactly what happens. Parmjit responds in line 2 with the second pair part *Yes please*, which is interpretable as the answer to the immediately prior question. Now consider the following:

1	Pam	Do you want to become a member?	[QUESTION A]
2	Steve	How much does it cost?	[QUESTION B]
3	Pam	Twenty pounds	[ANSWER B]
4	Steve	I don't think so	[ANSWER A]

This sequence begins like the previous one, with a question. Now, according to the characteristics set out above, a first pair part question should be followed by a second pair part answer, and this should be adjacent. However, this is not what occurs. In this instance, Pam's opening question in line 1 is not followed by the expected answer in line 2, but by a question *How much does it cost?* This so-called request for clarification is, clearly, directed back to Pam, and therefore it is appropriate that she should speak next. This she does in line 3, providing the answer *Twenty pounds* to the immediately prior question. Steve then takes up the next turn at talk in line 4 with *I don't think so*. This final utterance is now interpretable as the second pair part answer to Pam's original opening question *Do you want to become a member?*

Conversational sequences such as these are quite common, eg, where a question is not followed by an answer, or where a greeting is not followed by a greeting. We must, therefore, replace the condition of adjacency with what is known as conditional relevance. In other words, the management of conversation can occur over a number of turns at talk and relevance does not dissipate until a second pair part is given. In other words, once a first pair part is uttered it becomes conditionally relevant that the other participant should produce the relevant second pair part, or give an explanation as to why it has not been produced. Failure to produce the relevant second pair part is noticeable to the conversational participants. In the last example above, it was conditionally relevant that Steve provide a second pair part answer (answer A) to Pam's original first pair part question (question A). This was, in fact, provided, but it was produced after two intervening turns at talk. The sequence of talk in lines 2–3 served to clarify certain facts and information before Steve was able to respond to Pam's original question. It is rather like an aside, where the conversational participants negotiate further before returning to the main theme. Such sequences are referred to as *insertion sequences*. A further example, incorporating a couple of insertion sequences, should make this clear:

1	Customer	Do you have a copy of *Creating*	
2		*Affluence* by Deepak Chopra?	[QUESTION A]
3	Librarian	By who?	[QUESTION B]
4	Customer	Deepak Chopra	[ANSWER B]
5	Librarian	I'll have a look	[HOLD]
6	Customer	Thanks	[ACCEPT]
7		(21.0)	
8	Librarian	Sorry, it's out	[ANSWER A]

In this extract, the customer speaks first in lines 1–2 by producing a first pair part utterance that is typed as a question *Do you have a copy of* Creating Affluence *by Deepak Chopra?* It is evident that the librarian has either not heard or not understood the customer, as she does not provide an expected second pair part answer to the question. Instead, she produces a request for clarification *By who?* in line 3. This question is the start of the first insertion sequence. This request for clarification is also a first pair part question and, as such, it requires a second pair part answer. The customer provides this answer in line 4 by repeating the name of the author *Deepak Chopra*. Subsequently, a second insertion sequence is commenced in line 5, with the librarian informing the customer *I'll have a look*. This type of utterance acts as a sort of 'time out' that puts the conversation on hold (see Levinson 1983, 304). The implication here is that the librarian is going to check if the book is available. This first pair part utterance is then followed by the second pair part utterance *Thanks* in line 6. This type of utterance is usually referred to as an accept, ie, the customer has acknowledged and accepted the signal that the conversation is about to be put temporarily on hold. There is then a gap of 21 seconds (line 7) while the librarian checks the book's availability. Eventually, in line 8, the librarian produces the utterance *Sorry, it's out*. This utterance can be seen to be the second pair part answer to the original first pair part question *Do you have a copy of* Creating Affluence *by Deepak Chopra?* Again, therefore, we see how this original question set up a conditional relevancy that an answer should be provided. Once more, rather than the answer being provided in an adjacent utterance, insertion sequences intervened before the expected answer was given. It should be clear that if the librarian had failed to provide this second pair part answer then this would have been noticeable to the customer.

The final example in this section demonstrates how conversational participants notice the absence of a relevant second pair part, and how explanations for their absence may be provided:

1	Judy	Hi	[GREETING]
2		(2.0)	
3		Hi	[GREETING]
4		(1.5)	
5		HELLO	[GREETING]
6	Jackie	Oh, sorry, I was day-dreaming	[ACCOUNT]

In line 1, Judy produces a first pair part greeting *Hi*. Now, we know that it is conditionally relevant that this particular first pair part also requires a greeting as a second pair part. However, this is not forthcoming and there is a pause of around 2.0 seconds duration (line 2). Judy then repeats her previous first pair part greeting in line 3. That she does so may be taken as evidence that the failure of Jackie to produce a recognisable second pair part is noticed. Again, however, Jackie fails to produce a relevant second pair part and there is a further pause of 1.5 seconds (line 4). Judy now increases the volume of her utterance and produces the more formal greeting *HELLO* in line 5. Again, this so-called upgrading of her talk can be seen as evidence that Jackie's failure to produce a relevant second pair part is noticed. Finally, in line 6, Jackie responds with *Oh, sorry, I was day-dreaming*. Now, this utterance is not a greeting and it is not, therefore, a relevant second pair part to the initial greeting in line 1. However, it is apparent that Jackie recognises that it is relevant that she should have provided a second pair part, as she provides an explanation, or account, as to why she did not do so. Because conversational participants provide explicit accounts for the absence of second pair parts this supports the view that adjacency pairs are a fundamental unit of conversation. It would appear that conversational participants orient themselves to these structures. There is also evidence that conversational participants orient themselves to a set of rules that govern the allocation of turns at talk in any conversational interaction. In the next section we turn our attention to this issue of how turns at talk are managed in real time.

Turn Allocation

Sacks *et al* (1974; 1978) have proposed a mechanism that accounts for the collaborative achievement of conversation with respect to the characteristics of conversation highlighted earlier, and which functions on a turn-by-turn basis. In this so-called local management system, turns at talk are made up of *turn-constructional units*. These are the various utterances that the current speaker makes, and they are generally syntactic units like noun phrase, verb phrase, and so on. They can also be identified by prosodic features such as pitch-height, tempo and loudness variations (Local *et al* 1986). Initially a speaker is assigned just one turn-constructional unit, although its length is largely under the speaker's own control owing to the flexibility of natural language syntax and prosody. The end of a turn-constructional unit is a possible point for participants to change over, ie, the current speaker becomes the current listener and the current listener becomes the current speaker. This is known as a *transition relevance place*. Consider the following extract from a conversation between two people, A and B:

1	A	So would you like to learn to be able to write letters to him?
2	B	I would
3	A	Right. (pause) Well, you've learnt such a lot of words
4		reading them that all we have to practise now is putting
5		them together into a letter, isn't it?
6	B	Yeah

The first thing to notice is that the length of the utterances varies considerably, from the single word acknowledgement *Yeah* in line 6 to the complex tag-question *Well, you've learnt such a lot of words reading them that all we have to practise now is putting them together into a letter, isn't it?* in lines 3–5. Let us analyse the conversation line by line. In line 1, A is the first to speak with an utterance made up of just one turn-constructional unit. This is in the form of a question *So would you like to learn to be able to write letters to him?* The end of this turn-constructional unit is a transition relevance place where the roles of speaker and listener can alternate. In fact the roles do reverse and A ceases to be the current speaker as B takes over as the current speaker in line 2. A is now, therefore, the current listener as B takes a turn at talk with the turn-constructional unit *I would*. Again, the end of this unit is a transition relevance place and the next turn at talk transfers back to A. This time, A's utterance is made up of two turn-constructional units (lines 3–5). The first turn-constructional unit is the single word acknowledgement *Right*. You will notice that this is followed by a pause. This pause marks a possible transition relevance place that signals that the turn at talk could transfer back to B at this point. However, B does not take up a turn at talk at this juncture, and so A continues with a second turn-constructional unit *Well, you've learnt such a lot of words reading them that all we have to practise now is putting them together into a letter, isn't it?* Once more, the end of this tag-question represents a transition relevance place, ie, a place where it is relevant that the roles of speaker and listener could reverse. Indeed, the roles are reversed as B takes up a turn at talk in line 6 with the single turn-constructional unit *Yeah*. All conversations can be progressively analysed in this way, in terms of turn-constructional units and transition relevance places. The above analysis is summarised below, with each turn-constructional unit [TCU] and transition relevance place [TRP] marked:

1 A   [TCU *So would you like to learn to be able to write letters to him?*] [TRP]

2 B   [TCU *I would*] [TRP]

3 A   [TCU *Right*] [TRP] [TCU *Well, you've learnt such a lot of*

4   *words reading them that all we have to practise now is*

5   *putting them together into a letter, isn't it?*] [TRP]

6 B   [TCU *Yeah*]

To summarise, we have seen how initially a speaker is assigned just one turn-constructional unit and that its length is largely under the speaker's own control owing to the flexibility of language. We have also seen how the end of a turn-constructional unit is a possible point for the conversational participants to change over, ie, the current speaker could stop speaking and the current listener could begin to talk and, thereby, become the next speaker. Finally, participants can change over at these so-called transition relevance places, but do not necessarily do so, nor do they have to do so. We will now look a little more closely at what determines whether or not transition will occur by considering some rules of turn allocation.

Rule 1: Current Speaker Selects the Next Speaker

Transition rules operate at transition relevance places (the rules that follow are adapted from Levinson, 1983, 298). The first rule recognises the fact that it is possible to indicate within a turn-constructional unit that at its end another person is invited to speak. That is to say, it is possible specifically to allocate a following turn. This is outlined as follows:

If the CURRENT SPEAKER selects the NEXT SPEAKER in their turn at talk, then the CURRENT SPEAKER must stop speaking and the selected speaker must speak next. The transition occurs at the first transition relevance place after the NEXT SPEAKER has been selected.

Let us investigate the application of this rule by considering an example in which the next speaker is selected by the use of their name. Look at the following two-line extract taken from a conversation between three people, Kathryn, Meera and Karen:

1 Kathryn   Where did you put it, Meera?
2 Meera   It's on the table

Starting from the beginning, Kathryn is the current speaker and she specifically selects the next speaker by appending her name to her utterance in line 1 *Where did you put it, Meera?* It is relevant, therefore, that Kathryn, as the current speaker, should stop speaking and Meera, the selected speaker, should speak next. According to Rule 1, Meera should speak at the first transition relevance place after she has been selected. This she does by uttering *It's on the table* in line 2, immediately after the transition relevance place following Kathryn's turn-constructional unit. Now, for example, if Karen were to have spoken next and not Meera, this would have been interpretable as a violation of the turn allocation procedure, and it is likely to have led to Kathryn intervening with something like, 'I was asking Meera'. In summary, if the current speaker selects the next speaker, then the current speaker must stop speaking and the selected speaker should speak next at the first transition relevance place at the end of the turn-constructional unit. The above analysis can be outlined diagrammatically as follows:

1 Kathryn   [TCU *Where did you put it, Meera?*] [TRP – Rule 1]
2 Meera   [TCU *It's on the table*]

A further example of the application of Rule 1 by naming the next speaker is provided in the following conversational extract:

1 Carol   John, did you have to go abroad?
2 John   I needed the money, didn't I Chris?
3 Chris   Give him a break

Again we see that the current speaker, Carol, selects the next speaker within her current turn at talk. She does this in line 1 by specifically naming the next speaker with *John, did you have to go abroad?* That the name *John* is tagged to the beginning of the utterance and not the end, as in the previous example, is irrelevant. What is relevant, however, is that Carol should stop speaking at the end of her turn-constructional unit and that John should speak next at the first available transition relevance place. This John does in line 2 with the utterance *I needed the money, didn't I Chris?* Now, this utterance also selects the next speaker by nominating Chris. Therefore, it is relevant that John should now stop speaking and that Chris, as the selected speaker, should speak at the next available transition relevance place. Indeed, this is what happens, as Chris takes up his turn at talk in line 3 with *Give him a break*. We can now summarise this analysis as follows:

1 Carol   [TCU *John, did you have to go abroad?*]   [TRP – Rule 1]
2 John   [TCU *I needed the money, didn't I Chris?*]   [TRP – Rule 1]
3 Chris   [TCU *Give him a break*]

We see once more that turns at talk may be specifically allocated within one's current turn at talk, and that a useful technique for doing so is to nominate one of the conversational participants. However, there are other means of selecting the next speaker in a conversation. For example, it is possible to select the next speaker through the use of certain questions. Consider the following extract from the same conversation between the three people, Kathryn, Meera and Karen:

1 Kathryn   That's a nice one, Meera
2 Meera   Sorry?
3 Kathryn   It's a nice car

In this brief sequence Kathryn first takes a turn at talk in line 1 by uttering *That's a nice one, Meera*. Under Rule 1 as described so far, this nomination specifically serves to allocate the next turn at talk to Meera. It would appear, however, that Meera has either not heard Kathryn properly or has not understood what she meant, as Meera responds in line 2 with *Sorry?* It is this request for clarification that specifically allocates the next turn at talk to Kathryn and not Karen. This is because it was Kathryn who first made the utterance *That's a nice one*. Consequently, the subsequent *Sorry?* is seen as being directed specifically towards Kathryn's immediately prior utterance. Accordingly, it is Kathryn who should speak next. In fact, this is exactly what happens, as Kathryn takes up her turn at talk in line 3 with the explanatory *It's a nice car*. This analysis is summarised below:

1 Kathryn   [TCU *That's a nice one, Meera*] [TRP – Rule 1]
2 Meera   [TCU *Sorry?*] [TRP – Rule 1]
3 Kathryn   [TCU *It's a nice car*]

A further, slightly longer, example of the use of questions to select the next speaker is drawn from the same three-participant conversation:

1 Meera   Mind you, it's not all that, Kathryn
2 Kathryn   What?
3 Meera   It's not all that, Kathryn
4 Kathryn   What do you mean?
5 Meera   It's not all that ... you know ... it's not fab

A similar analysis may be made of this extract to the previous one. At the beginning it is Meera who is the current speaker. She takes a turn at talk in line 1 with the turn-constructional unit *Mind you, it's not all that, Kathryn*. This utterance again specifically allocates the next turn at talk to Kathryn by nominating her. It is relevant that Meera should stop speaking and that Kathryn should speak next. This Kathryn does in line 2 with the query *What?* As before, this query is interpretable as being specifically directed towards Meera and not Karen, as it was Meera who made the immediately prior utterance. This query, therefore, serves specifically to allocate the next turn at talk to Meera. Meera does indeed take up the talk at the next available transition relevance place, and responds in line 3 with a part-repetition of her previous utterance *It's not all that, Kathryn*. The fact that Meera partially repeats her previous utterance suggests that Meera has interpreted Kathryn's query as a signal that Kathryn did not fully hear her comment. Again, Meera's line 3 utterance specifically selects the next speaker as Kathryn, and it is once more relevant that Meera should stop speaking and that Kathryn should speak next. Kathryn does speak next in line 4 but, again, she responds with a query. This time it is the more specific *What do you mean?* The fact that Kathryn's response is an expansion of her previous *What?* suggests that it was not the case that she did not hear Meera's previous comment, but that she did not understand it. This question again serves to select the next speaker as

Meera, and not Karen, and so Kathryn stops speaking and Meera takes up the talk at the next available transition relevance place in line 5 with the explanatory *It's not all that … you know … it's not fab*. This analysis may be summarised as follows:

1 Meera   [TCU *Mind you, it's not all that, Kathryn*]
            [TRP – Rule 1]
2 Kathryn   [TCU *What?*] [TRP – Rule 1]
3 Meera   [TCU *It's not all that, Kathryn*] [TRP – Rule 1]
4 Kathryn   [TCU *What do you mean?*] [TRP – Rule 1]
5 Meera   [TCU *it's not all that … you know … it's not fab*]

Rule 2: Next Speaker Self-Selects

So far, we have considered only examples where the current speaker selects the next speaker within their turn at talk, either by nominating the person or by using specific questions. However, there will always be instances when the current speaker does not select the next speaker. In instances such as these, any participant in the conversation may self-select themselves as the next speaker. Usually, it is the first person to speak who gains the right to the next turn at talk. This rule of turn allocation may be stated as follows:

If the CURRENT SPEAKER does not select the NEXT SPEAKER in their turn at talk, then any other person may self-select themselves as the NEXT SPEAKER. The first person to speak gains the right to the next turn.

Consider the following extract:

1 Karen   So that's what happened
2 Kathryn   Have you seen that film, Meera?
3 Meera   No

In this sequence, Karen, as the current speaker in line 1, does not specifically select the next speaker during her turn-constructional unit. As a consequence, any participant has the right to claim the next turn at talk. In this instance it is Kathryn who speaks first in line 2. She therefore claims the right to the next turn at talk by uttering *Have you seen that film, Meera?* Interestingly, Kathryn subsequently nominates the next speaker during her turn-constructional unit, ie, Meera. Therefore, it is relevant under Rule 1 that Meera should speak next, which she does in line 3 with the answer *No*. In summary, we see how the current speaker, Karen, chooses not to select the next speaker in the conversation and how Kathryn claims the right to the next turn at talk by speaking up first at the transition relevance place at the end of Karen's turn-constructional unit. The above analysis may be summarised as follows:

1 Karen   [TCU *So that's what happened*] [TRP – Rule 2]
2 Kathryn [TCU *Have you seen that film, Meera?*] [TRP – Rule 1]
3 Meera   [TCU *No*]

A further example should make the application of this turn allocation rule clearer. Consider the following extract from the same conversation:

1 Kathryn Well, I thought the Brit Awards were brill
2   (pause)
3 Karen   David's coming tomorrow
4 Meera   Did you miss him?
5 Karen   Yeah

Once again, Kathryn speaks first in line 1 with an utterance made up of just one turn-constructional unit *Well, I thought the Brit Awards were brill*. It is evident that she does not select the next speaker within this turn. Consequently, Rule 1 does not apply, but Rule 2 comes into play. We know that, under Rule 2, if the current speaker does not select the next speaker then any other person may self-select themselves as the next speaker. There is actually a slight pause in line 2 after Kathryn's utterance, but then Karen speaks first in line 3. She has self-selected herself as the next speaker and the turn at talk transfers to her. Karen's utterance is also made up of just one turn-constructional unit *David's coming tomorrow*. Once more we see that, like Kathryn before her, she has not selected the next speaker within her turn. Again, therefore, Rule 1 does not apply and Rule 2 comes into play once more. As a consequence, any other person in the conversation can self-select themselves as the next speaker, with the one who speaks first gaining the right to the next turn. In this instance, it is Meera who speaks first in line 4 with the utterance *Did you miss him?* Now, this utterance is framed as a question and it can be seen as being specifically directed to Karen, as it was Karen who had made the immediately prior utterance. In this instance, therefore, Rule 1 has come back into play, as the current speaker has selected the next speaker. It is relevant, therefore, that Meera should stop speaking at the end of her turn-constructional unit and that the selected speaker should speak at the first available transition relevance place. We see that Rule 1 is, in fact, followed and that Karen speaks next in line 5 with the affirmation *Yeah*. This analysis may be summarised as follows:

1	Kathryn	[TCU *Well, I thought the Brit Awards were brill*]
2		[TRP – Rule 2]
3	Karen	[TCU *David's coming tomorrow*] [TRP – Rule 2]
4	Meera	[TCU *did you miss him?*] [TRP – Rule 1]
5	Karen	[TCU *yeah*]

To summarise, we have seen how the end of a turn-constructional unit is a possible point for conversational participants to change over, ie, for the current speaker to become a current listener and a current listener to become the current speaker. So far, we have examined two means of managing this transition: (1) by selecting the next speaker under Rule 1, and (2) by a conversational participant self-selecting themselves under Rule 2. We have noted, however, that while conversational participants may alter roles at these so-called transition relevance places, they do not necessarily do so, nor do they have to do so. In order to explain turn allocation in instances where neither the next speaker is selected nor anyone self-selects themselves as the next speaker we must invoke another rule.

Rule 3: Current Speaker Continues

Consider the following, taken from our ongoing conversation between Kathryn, Meera and Karen:

1	Karen	It was all a bit quick
2		(pause)
3	Karen	Anyway, I took it home with me

We see that Karen has not selected the next speaker within her first turn-constructional unit in line 1 *It was all a bit quick*. Therefore, Rule 1 does not apply. Rule 2 would now come into play, ie, any conversational participant could self-select themselves as the next speaker. The transition relevance place for this is marked by the pause in line 2 following Karen's first utterance. However, neither of the other two conversational participants self-selects herself: neither Kathryn nor Meera speaks. Recall that we noted that transition can take place at the end of a turn-constructional unit, but that it does not have to do so. Consequently, as no other participant self-selects herself as the next speaker, Karen claims a right to a further turn-constructional unit and she continues after the pause in line 3 with *Anyway, I took it home with me*. The rule governing this situation is set out as follows:

If the CURRENT SPEAKER has not selected the NEXT SPEAKER, and no other person self-selects themselves as NEXT SPEAKER, then the CURRENT SPEAKER may continue to talk, but need not do so.

The foregoing analysis may be summarised as follows:

1 Karen   [TCU *It was all a bit quick*]
2   [TRP – Rule 3]
3 Karen   [TCU *Anyway, I took it home with me*]

Another example should make this clearer. Consider the following extract from a conversation, again between three people:

1 Jane   Anyway, that's what I think
2   (pause)
3   I could be wrong
4   (pause)
5   I don't have a strong view
6 Anne   Mm
7 Sue   Yeah

In this extract it is Jane who speaks first in line 1 with the utterance *Anyway, that's what I think*. The transition relevance place subsequent to this single turn-constructional unit is marked by the immediately following pause in line 2. This is a place where the turn at talk could alternate to one of the other participants. As Jane has not selected the next speaker within her turn, Rule 1 does not apply. Rule 2 would then come into play. However, neither Anne nor Sue self-select themselves as the next speaker and so Rule 3 now comes into play. According to this rule, as Jane did not select the next speaker, and as no other participant self-selected themselves as next speaker, Jane can claim rights to a further turn-constructional unit. This is exactly what Jane does and she speaks next in line 3 with *I could be wrong*. Once more this utterance is made up of just the one turn-constructional unit, and the transition relevance place is again marked by the subsequent pause in line 4. It is evident that Jane's line 3 utterance *I could be wrong* again does not select the next speaker and so Rule 1 does not apply. Rule 2 therefore comes into play again. However, once more, neither Anne nor Sue self-select themselves as the next speaker. So, again, Rule 3 is applied and Jane continues with her talk by claiming the rights to yet another turn-constructional unit in line 5 with *I don't have a strong view*. This final utterance by Jane again does not select the next speaker and so Rule 1 cannot apply. This time, however, Anne self-selects herself as the next speaker under Rule 2 by speaking first in line 6 with the token *Mm*. This utterance similarly does not select the next speaker under Rule 1, but Sue can be seen to self-select herself as the next speaker under Rule 2 by speaking up first in line 7 with the token *Yeah*. This analysis may be summarised as follows:

1	Jane	[TCU *Anyway, that's what I think*]
2		[TRP – Rule 3]
3		[TCU *I could be wrong*]
4		[TRP – Rule 3]
5		[TCU *I don't have a strong view*] [TRP – Rule 2]
6	Anne	[TCU *Mm*] [TRP – Rule 2]
7	Sue	[TCU *Yeah*]

Rule 4: Recursive Application of Rules 1–3

In the above analysis we have seen that when Rule 3 has been applied, ie, the current speaker chooses to continue with their turn at talk because they have not selected the next speaker and no other speaker has self-selected themselves as the next speaker, then the three rules operate recursively at every subsequent transition relevance place. To reiterate, we saw how Jane continued with her turn at talk in line 3 with the utterance *I could be wrong* as a consequence of the application of Rule 3. At the transition relevance place marked by the end of this turn-constructional unit (line 4), all three rules were once more applied. We first considered whether or not Rule 1 was applicable, ie, did Jane select the next speaker? The answer is, of course, no. We then considered Rule 2, ie, did any other conversational participant self-select themselves as the next speaker? Again, the answer is no. We finally considered Rule 3, ie, in the absence of Jane selecting the next speaker and no other participant self-selecting herself as the next speaker, did Jane continue? The answer to this is yes. She continued with her talk in line 5 with *I don't have a strong view*. We continue with our analysis in just this way at every available transition relevance place. The next one in the current sequence occurs at the end of Jane's line 5 utterance *I don't have a strong view*. Again we consider the application of each rule at this transition relevance place. Does Rule 1 apply? No. Does Rule 2 apply? Yes. It applies because Anne self-selects herself as the next speaker by speaking first in line 6 with the token *Mm*. Thus, after a series of three turns at talk by Jane (lines 1, 3 and 5), speaker change is eventually effected in line 6 by Anne taking up the talk. Consequently, we see how Rules 1–3 are applied recursively at every available transition relevance place until a change is effected from one speaker to another. This management procedure may be summarised as follows:

When Rule 3 has been selected by the CURRENT SPEAKER, then Rules 1–3 apply at the next transition relevance place, and recursively at the next transition relevance place, until speaker change is effected.

Overlapping Talk

We have noted that a general characteristic of conversation is that conversational participants talk one at a time. Clearly, however, there will be instances when this is not so. For example, a listener may begin their talk before the current speaker has finished speaking and overlap the speaker. During such instances, the overlapping talk is noticeable as such and the conversational participants attempt to rectify the situation by reverting to a state of one, and only one, speaker as quickly as possible. The explanation for this return to one-at-a-time talk is that participants generally cannot process information from more than one source at a time, and that much of the overlapping talk cannot be heard (Edelsky, 1981). It is apparent that some overlapping talk is considered to be accidental, while other overlaps are viewed as wilful interruptions. How can we explain these perceived differences? Well, the answer lies once again in a consideration of the application of the rules of turn allocation. We will now consider examples of these two types of overlapping talk which are known respectively as (1) inadvertent overlap, and (2) violative interruption.

Inadvertent Overlap

Consider the following extract from a conversation between two people (NB: the symbol consisting of two parallel lines // indicates the starting point at which the talk is overlapped by the talk on the immediately following line:)

1   Deepak   You've done that before ... // haven't you?
2   Andy   Yeah

In this brief extract it is Deepak who speaks first in line 1. Notice that his utterance is framed as a tag-question, ie, he appends the tag *haven't you?* to the end of his statement *You've done that before*. Now, tag-questions are especially prone to being overlapped because they are often spoken with a slight pause between the main body of the utterance and the tag itself. This is the case with Deepak's utterance: he makes a slight pause after *You've done that before* prior to appending the tag *haven't you?* It should be apparent from our foregoing discussion of turn allocation that a current listener in a conversation is constantly monitoring the talk of the current speaker for upcoming transition relevance places. That is to say, a current listener is attempting to determine those places where it is relevant and appropriate that the roles of speaker and listener should alternate. Conversationalists are clearly extremely skilled in doing this, as we have already noted that the transition from one speaker to another is so swift that it has to be measured in microseconds. Consequently, returning to our example, the slight pause after Deepak's statement *You've done that before* can be seen as signalling a possible transition relevance place. It is, therefore, a potentially relevant place at which the listener can take up a turn at talk. In fact this is what Andy does in line 2, with the confirmation *Yeah*. However, Deepak evidently did not intend this slight pause to represent a transition relevance place, as he continued by adding the tag *haven't you?* Thus, Andy's line 2 utterance *Yeah* overlaps some of Deepak's talk. However, this type of overlapping talk is accidental or inadvertent. In other words, there was no intention on the part of the listener to wilfully interrupt the speaker. The overlapping talk occurred because, in this instance, the current listener misjudged an upcoming transition relevance place. Now consider the following extract of a conversation between three people:

1 Daniel   I shouldn't have started
2 Anna   // Get away
3 Chris   No way

In line 1, Daniel opens with the statement *I shouldn't have started*. This turn-constructional unit does not select the next speaker under Rule 1 and so Rule 2 comes into play. That is to say, either of the other two conversational participants can self-select themselves as the next speaker. It is apparent from the extract that both Anna and Chris attempt to self-select themselves as the next speaker. What has happened in this instance, however, is that they have both spoken at the same time. Consequently, their utterances overlap (lines 2 and 3). Again, however, we can see that this was not a wilful attempt to interrupt Daniel, as their contributions came at an appropriate transition relevance place at the end of Daniel's turn-constructional unit. The overlap was simply a case of two speakers both starting their talk at the same time. Again, therefore, from an understanding of the rules of turn allocation we can see that this is another case of inadvertent overlap.

Violative Interruption
Now contrast the previous example with the following extract taken from a conversation between two people:

```
1   Nicholas   I thought it was a sensible consi//deration to walk
2   Mary                                    That's stupid because
3              no one can make those sorts of decisions any more
```

In this extract, first look at where Mary's talk in lines 2–3 occurs. It can be seen to begin on the third syllable of the word *consideration* currently being spoken by Nicholas in line 1. It should be apparent that the middle of a word is not a transition relevance place and, therefore, not an appropriate point for the turn at talk to alternate. We have already made clear that the rules of turn allocation operate at transition relevance places. Consequently, if any conversational participant seeks to apply these rules at any place in the conversation other than a transition relevance place, this will be noticeable as a violation of the turn allocation procedure. The fact that Mary's turn at talk does not begin at an appropriate transition relevance place is perceived as a violation of the rules of turn allocation. Her talk is perceived as a wilful interruption and not an inadvertent overlap. A further example should help to make this concept clear:

```
1   Amanda    Mind you, I would
2             never have //gone so far ...
3   Kevin              // Like heck
4   Hilary                 Oh::::::::: I bet
```

In lines 1–2 Amanda is engaged in a stretch of talk *Mind you, I would never have gone so far ...* This proposition is incomplete as it is overlapped, commencing on the word *gone* in line 2. Interestingly, Amanda's talk is overlapped by both Kevin and Hilary simultaneously. However, the point at which they overlap Amanda's talk does not occur at a legitimate transition relevance place. The only appropriate transition relevance place occurs at the very end of Amanda's utterance, but her talk is overlapped at the juncture between the words *have* and *gone*. Now, clearly, this overlap cannot be analysed as being inadvertent as the juncture between an auxiliary verb (*have*) and a lexical verb (*gone*) can never be a transition relevance place. It is not possible to argue, therefore, that Kevin and Hilary have misjudged a potential upcoming transition relevance place. Therefore, this overlap is analysable as a violative interruption that wilfully ignores the rules of turn allocation in conversations. A further interesting point in this example is that because both Kevin and Hilary overlap Amanda at the same time, their own talk overlaps the other's. Consequently, Kevin's line 3 *Like heck* is overlapped by Hilary's line 4 *Oh I bet*. Now, this particular overlapping talk is actually inadvertent overlap. In other words, both Kevin and Hilary, despite violating the rules of turn allocation, both self-selected themselves as next speaker (interrupter) at precisely the same time. Consequently, there is an accidental overlap of Kevin and Hilary's talk. A final point to note is that there appears to be some recognition from Hilary that her line 4 utterance has indeed inadvertently overlapped Kevin's talk because she prolongs the single vowel vocalisation *Oh* (as denoted in the text by the sequence of colons). This prolongation continues until Kevin's line 3 utterance is completed and then, at this point, Hilary completes her own initiation of a turn at talk with *I bet*. This brief example demonstrates very well how conversational participants manage conversations on a turn-by-turn basis and how they can time and implement their contributions both rapidly and accurately.

To summarise, inadvertent overlaps typically occur at possible transition relevance places. They often occur because one or more of the conversational participants perceives an upcoming transition relevance place where the speaker may not have intended there to be one. Alternatively, they occur because more than one person attempts to self-select themselves as the next speaker at an appropriate transition relevance place. In contrast, violative interruptions can be seen as transgressions of the rules of turn allocation. As such, they typically occur where there is no valid transition relevance place.

Resolving Overlapping Talk

We have already noted that in the relatively few instances when there is overlapping talk, conversational participants attempt to rectify the situation by reverting to a state of one, and only one, speaker as quickly as possible. How do they achieve this? Well, there are two main strategies: (1) dropping out, and (2) competitive allocation. We will consider each of these below.

Dropping Out

We have already witnessed one example of dropping out in the last example above. We noted that Amanda appeared to be engaged in an ongoing stretch of talk, and that both Kevin and Hilary interrupted her. It is evident that, as they speak, Amanda drops out: her talk tails away in line 2 with *never have gone so far* ... As Amanda drops out, so Kevin and Hilary continue with their talk, although theirs is a violative interruption. A further example of dropping out is provided in the following extract from a conversation between three people:

1 Dale He'll have to sing a lot better
2 Krishna // He was trying ...
3 Jean He never really had the opportunity to show how good he was

In line 1, Dale does not select the next speaker under Rule 1. Consequently, any conversational participant could self-select themselves as the next speaker under Rule 2. Again, we see that, at the appropriate transition relevance place at the end of Dale's line 1 turn-constructional unit, both Krishna and Jean attempt to self-select themselves as the next speaker. They both attempt to take up their turn at talk at the same time and so their utterances overlap in lines 2 and 3. This is another example of inadvertent overlap. However, in this instance, we see that Krishna drops out and thereby relinquishes his claim to a turn at talk. Jean, therefore, continues with her turn.

Competitive Allocation

In contrast to the examples of dropping out highlighted above, not all speakers are as willing to relinquish their turn at talk. In these instances there occurs what is known as *competitive allocation*. That is to say, one or more of the conversational participants competes either to retain their turn at talk or to take over the turn at talk. Consider the following, taken again from the conversation between Nicholas and Mary:

1 Nicholas that way I de//cided TO KEEP THE MONEY TO MYSELF
2 Mary But you ...

As in the previous example drawn from this conversation, Mary once more attempts a violative interruption by trying to take a turn at talk at a point where there is no appropriate transition relevance place. She attempts to begin her talk in line 2 within the second syllable of the word *decided* being spoken by Nicholas in line 1. However, on this occasion, Nicholas is unwilling to drop out. He therefore competes to retain his turn by upgrading his talk. He does this by increasing his volume and continuing to speak. This has the effect of overriding Mary and she can be seen to drop out in line 2, almost before she has got started. Increasing the volume of one's talk is a frequent method of upgrading. Further strategies include slowing the rate of speech, lengthening the vowel sounds and accompanying the talk with non-verbal gestures, such as raising a hand or a finger. These non-verbal accompaniments act as holding devices that serve to indicate to the person who is attempting to interrupt that the current speaker is not yet ready to relinquish their turn. Competitive allocation must not necessarily always occur at moments of violative interruption, however. Consider the following example of inadvertent overlap.

1	Paul	can you help with the map reading or not?
2	Craig	// Yes … erm … but …
3	John	Yeah BUT I CAN'T GET THERE by myself you know

It is evident that Craig and John's overlapping talk in lines 2 and 3 is inadvertent because it can be seen to occur at the transition relevance place at the end of Paul's line 1 question *Can you help with the map reading or not?* Again, this is an instance where two conversational participants have both attempted to self-select themselves as the next speaker, under Rule 2, at the same time. As they both begin their talk, Craig appears to be more hesitant in line 2, with his *Yes … erm … but …* John, however, is less indecisive and he upgrades his talk by increasing his volume for part of his line 3 utterance, ie, *BUT I CAN'T GET THERE*. Once it is apparent that Craig has dropped out, John reduces his volume to a normal conversational level again as he completes his utterance with *by myself you know*. In this instance, it can be seen that the competitive allocation procedure has worked to resolve the overlapping talk in a relatively short time. In fact, this is true of most attempts to resolve overlapping talk, ie, it is typically resolved quickly with only a small number of words being overlapped. A final point worth considering is in relation to our earlier comment that overlapping talk potentially cannot be heard properly. We are aware that a characteristic of collaborative conversation is that the current speaker strives to ensure that they are being attended to, understood and, therefore, heard. How does a speaker who has had part of his or her talk overlapped by another ensure that important information has been heard properly? Well, the most common method is recycling.

Recycling

Consider yet another example of inadvertent overlap in a three-participant conversation. (NB: the asterisk * indicates the point at which the overlapping talk ceases:)

1 Lynn So what's the problem?
2 Richie // You could have... *
3 Emma Lisa's the pro ... * Lisa's the problem as far as I can see

In line 1 Lynn does not select the next speaker under Rule 1. Consequently, either Richie or Emma may self-select themselves as the next speaker under Rule 2. In fact, they both attempt to take up the next turn at talk at the same time and there is an inadvertent overlap. We see that Richie's incomplete line 2 utterance *You could have* is overlapped by Emma's self-edited line 3 utterance *Lisa's the pro ...* It is evident that Richie then drops out in line 2 as he relinquishes the turn at talk to Emma. Subsequently, as Emma continues with her turn at talk she recycles that part of her utterance that has been overlapped, ie, *Lisa's the problem*, before completing her utterance with *as far as I can see*. The effect of this is to re-present the information that may have been obscured, and therefore unheard, because of the overlap. A final example should make recycling clear:

1 Valerie Well ... I think you should a//pologise as* soon ...
2 Graham   Oh give up
3 Valerie YOU SHOULD APOLOgise as soon as possible

This sequence is another example of violative interruption. This is evidenced by the fact that Graham's *Oh give up* overlaps Valerie's line 1 utterance on the second syllable of the word *apologise*. This is clearly not a valid transition relevance place and the talk, therefore, violates the rules of turn allocation. As Graham's overlapping talk may have obscured the hearing of Valerie's line 1 proposition, she recycles a substantial part of the utterance in line 3 when Graham's violative interruption has terminated. Interestingly, Valerie also upgrades her recycled talk in line 3 by increasing the volume. As she already has the floor, this may be intended to prevent Graham making a further bid to interrupt. It is also possible, however, that the increased volume is intended to stress the emphatic nature of her proposition. It is not possible to determine the speaker's rationale in a situation like this. All we can do is observe that Valerie recycled talk that was made potentially unhearable by a violative interruption, and that she upgraded this talk when she had regained her turn at talk. As we have seen, recycling is not used in every instance of overlapping talk, but it is a readily available technique for conversational participants to use if they consider that important pieces of information may have been distorted by the noise of overlapping talk.

This concludes our discussion of conversation. To summarise, in this chapter we have seen that conversations are highly coordinated, collaborative social events and that while there is no predetermined cognitive map that dictates their form, nevertheless, they are highly structured. This structure has been explained in terms of a fundamental unit of conversation known as the adjacency pair. We have noted that these ordered adjacency pairs are produced by different speakers and that they are typed so that a particular first pair part requires a particular second pair part. However, through an examination of actual sequences of talk we recognised the need to replace the condition of adjacency with the concept of conditional relevance. The so-called local management of conversations has also been explored and explained in terms of a set of four rules that govern how turns at talk are allocated to conversational participants in real time. Turns at talk are seen to alternate legitimately only at so-called transition relevance places. We noted early in the chapter that a general feature of conversation is that only one participant talks at any one time. However, we also recognised that there will always be instances when this is not so. This phenomenon of overlapping talk was investigated through an application of the rules of turn allocation. The exploration led us to identify some types of overlap as inadvertent and others as violative. Inadvertent overlap was seen to occur when one or more of the conversational participants perceived an upcoming transition relevance place where the current speaker did not intend there to be one. Violative interruption, on the other hand, was identified as a wilful transgression of the rules of turn allocation, typically occurring at a juncture where there can be no valid transition relevance place. We concluded the chapter by considering two main strategies by which any overlapping talk, inadvertent or violative, may be resolved. The first is known as dropping out, in which one of the overlapped participants simply relinquishes their attempt to take a turn at talk. The second is competitive allocation, in which an overlapped participant upgrades their talk by, for example, increasing their volume and slowing the rate of their speech. Therefore, rather than relinquishing their attempt to take a turn at talk they actively compete for a turn. Finally, we saw how a speaker whose talk had been overlapped, and therefore potentially unheard, may redeliver the utterance either in part or in whole. We referred to this management strategy as recycling.

We began this book by outlining the nature of human communication and highlighting language and speech as the major facets. In subsequent chapters we have explored some of the theory that allows an understanding of these areas. We have considered the key properties of language, its acquisition and its development. We have taken a considerable amount of time to examine how the meaning units that we call words are constructed and strung together to create purposeful utterances. Some of the aspects of the social use of language have also been considered, and how language may be varied according to the environmental context. We have also thought carefully about the production of English speech sounds and how these may also be systematically combined. We have considered a variety of processes that may affect the articulation of sounds in isolated words and in the continuous stream of spoken words that we call connected speech. In this, our final chapter, we have considered the management of participation in the most consummate of human communicative behaviours, conversation. It is my hope that this brief introduction has illuminated this fascinating topic and that it might encourage you to investigate further why and how, of all the creatures upon this planet, we are the most compulsive of communicators.

Revision Exercises

9.1 List three characteristics of conversation.

9.2 Identify the turn-constructional units [TCU] and transition relevance places [TRP] in the following extract from a conversation between two people, A and B:

1 A He shows his fist to you does he?
2 B Yeah (…) he smoking all the time
3 A He's smoking all the time
4 B Yeah
5 A Yeah I know (…) but tell him off

9.3 In each of the following three conversational extracts determine whether the overlapping talk is inadvertent or violative:

A 1 Li Wei   Of course the most pre//ssing issue for
  2 Lisa   Can't you just decide
  3   (.) it's driving me mad thinking about it

B: 1 Josie: I think they tried it (.) //or something like it
   2 Sheilah: Yes they did

C: 1 Carl: This meeting's over
   2 Joe: //Surely not
   3 Rob: It can't be

Activities

9.4 Make a 15-minute audio tape recording of an informal conversation between three adult friends who know each other well. Transcribe the conversation turn by turn, marking pauses and overlaps. Use the following key to mark pauses:

(..)   brief pause (>0.5 sec, <1 sec)
(…)   pause (>1 sec, <1.5 sec)
(2.0) longer pause in seconds, eg, (2.5), (4.0), (6.0)

In addition, use the standard notation of two parallel lines // to indicate the starting point at which talk on one line is overlapped by the talk on the immediately following line.

Analyse the transcription and determine all instances of overlapping talk. What is their frequency of occurrence? Do you consider this to be high or is this phenomenon relatively rare? Are the overlaps predominantly inadvertent or violative? Attempt an explanation of any overlaps in terms of the rules of turn allocation and the projection of upcoming transition relevance places. Are any violative interruptions performed by just one participant or distributed evenly among all participants? How do you explain these findings? Now investigate how the participants resolve any overlapping talk. Is there a preferred strategy? Does dropping out or competitive allocation prevail? Can you explain why? Are there any instances of recycling? Finally, consider whether or not your findings would have been different if you had made a recording of a conversation between three people who had never met before? How might your findings have been different if the conversation were more formal, eg, a couple meeting with a bank manager for the purpose of securing a loan?

9.5 Observe several children of different ages playing with their peers (eg, 2-year-olds, 3-year-olds, 4-year-olds, and so on). Do the children demonstrate characteristics of adult-type conversations (eg, turn-taking, collaboration, resolving overlapping talk), or do they, for example, talk in monologues either to themselves or at another child? Do all age groups demonstrate the same types of 'conversational' skills? What are the differences between the age groups? At what age do you consider that children are able to engage in conversation? How do you explain this?

Key to Exercises

1.1 Language is the ability to understand and use symbols (words); speech is the transmission system of language, and non-verbal communication is the systematic and non-systematic way in which human beings transmit meaning to one another other than by spoken language.

1.2 Any three of the following prerequisites for language development: an understanding of cause and effect; reciprocity; symbolic understanding; memory. Any three of the following prerequisites for speech development: an ability to produce a range of sounds; hearing and listening skills; imitation; motivation.

1.3 Production, transmission and reception.

1.4 The process that takes place at the linguistic level of the agent is the encoding of thoughts into linguistic symbols, and at the linguistic level of the recipient it is the decoding of these linguistic symbols.

2.1 Any five of the following: arbitrariness, duality, systematicity, structure-dependence, productivity, displacement, specialisation, cultural transmission.

2.2 *Langage* refers to the possession of a general language capacity. *Langue* refers to any particular world language. As we require *langage* in order to acquire a particular *langue*, we may say that *langage* comes first.

2.3 *knife* and *fork*
     cup and *spoon*
     black and *coffee* (ie, *black coffee*)

2.4

I	*like*	*cheese*			= 3
my	*mum*	*play*			= 3
where	*daddy*				= 2
kick	*ball*				= 2
Harry					= 1
see	*my*	*mum*	*play*	*ball*	= 5
				TOTAL =	16
				MLU =	16/6
				=	2.7

We know that the child is 3;04 years old and, from Table 2.2, we know that the MLU for a child of this age should be between 3.47 and 3.78. As this child has an MLU of 2.7 this is clearly less than expected and it is not, therefore, age appropriate. Note, however, that this assessment has been based on only six utterances and the findings should be treated with caution.

3.1 An open word class is one that can be expanded indefinitely by the addition of new words. In contrast, a closed word class cannot be expanded, ie, it has a fixed number of words that constitute the class.

3.2 *his*(F) *dis-*(B)*interest*(F) *show*(F)-*ed*(B) *when*(F) *I*(F) *re-*(B)*play*(F)-*ed*(B)
     the(F) *sing*(F)-*ing*(B) *detective*(F) *video*(F)-*s*(B)
     if(F) *you*(F) *re-*(B)*consider*(F) *I*(F) *will*(F) *happy*(F)-*ly*(B) *provide*(F)
     some(F) *in-*(B)*expensive*(F) *watch*(F)-*es*(B)
     the(F) *priest*(F)-*s*(B) *determine*(F)-*ed*(B) *that*(F) *their*(F) *life*(F)-*s*(B)
     were(F) *pre-*(B)*ordain*(F)-*ed*(B)

3.3 *she* (det) *drank* (verb) *the* (det) *red* (adj) *liquid* (noun) *quickly* (adv) *yesterday* (adv), *Margaret* (noun) *gave* (verb) *it* (pron) *to* (prep) *him* (pron) *three* (num) *men* (noun) *cried* (verb) *because* (conj) *they* (pron) *were* (verb) *very* (adv) *unhappy* (adj)

the (det) *furry* (adj) *cat* (noun) *jumped* (verb) *in* (prep) *the* (det) *large* (adj) *yellow* (adj) *box* (noun)

the (det) *first* (num) *girl* (noun) *and* (conj) *her* (pron) *friend* (noun) *left* (verb) *for* (prep) *home* (noun)

quietly (adv), *quietly* (adv), *the* (det) *little* (adj) *mouse* (noun) *crept* (verb)

the (det) *right* (adj) *man* (noun)

a (det) *man* (noun) *on* (prep) *the* (det) *right* (noun)

may (verb) *I* (pron) *be* (verb) *the* (det) *first* (num) *to congratulate* (verb) *you* (pron)

4.1 Syntax refers to the rules that govern the combination of words and their sequential placement, in order to create meaningful grammatical phrases and clauses.

4.2

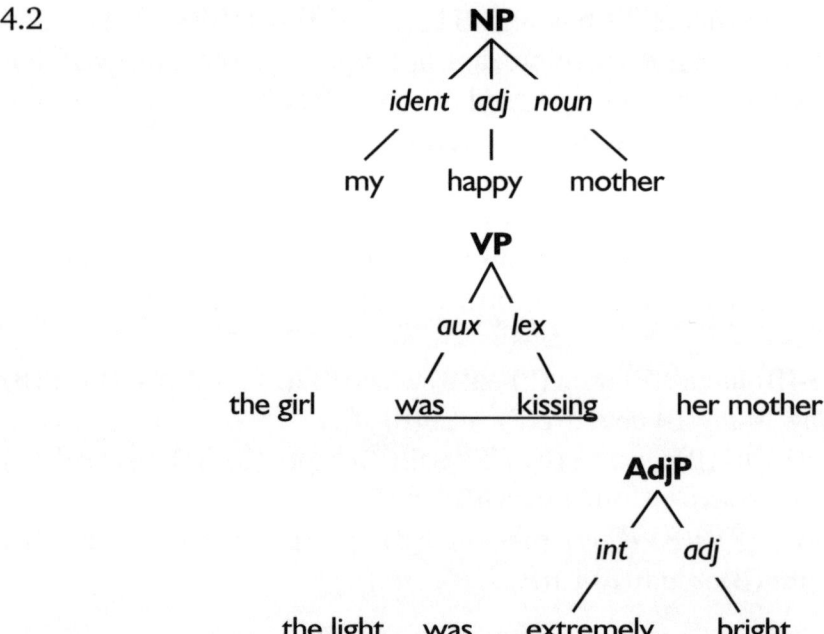

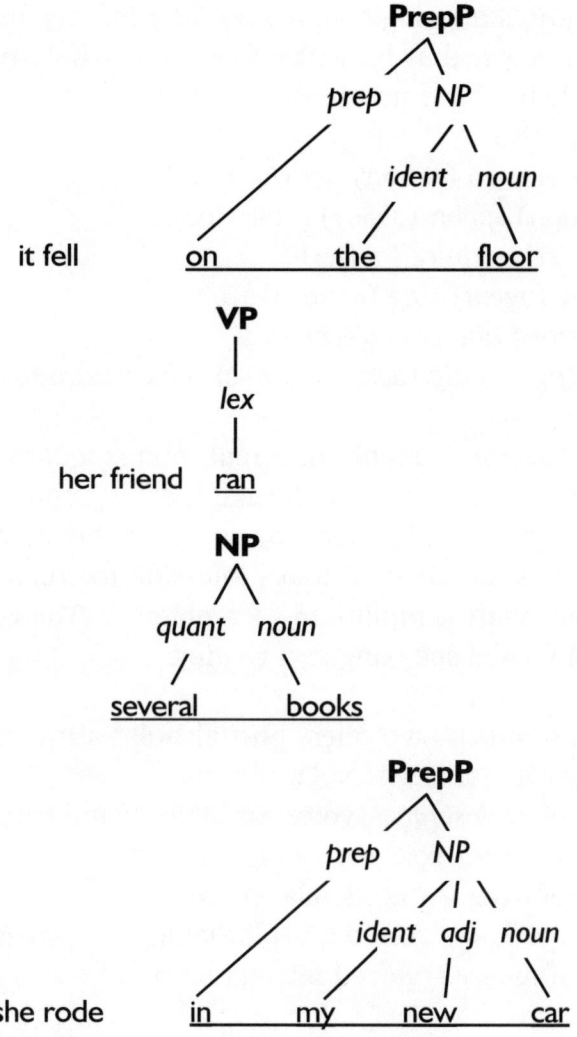

4.3 *his sister* (S:NP) *called* (V:VP) *his mother* (O:NP)
 Lucy (S:NP) *played* (V:VP) *happily* (A:AdvP)
 Margaret (S:NP) *gave* (V:VP) *Graham* (O$_i$:NP) *a Valentine card* (O$_d$:NP)
 the dog (S:NP) *barked* (V:VP)
 your mother (S:NP) *sent* (V:VP) *a letter* (O:NP)
 Adele (S:NP) *was* (V:VP) *reluctant* (C:AdjP)
 the two therapists (S:NP) *taught* (V:VP) *the child* (O:NP) *in Darlington*
   (A:PrepP)
 the song (S:NP) *made* (V:VP) *Kathryn* (O:NP) *happy* (C:AdjP)

5.1 Holophrases are single words used by infants, usually up to the age of 2;00 years, that have the force of a whole phrase which would normally be made up of several adult words.

5.2 *ball* (*object*) *go* (*action*) *net* (*location*)
hit (*action*) *spoon* (*object*) *table* (*location*)
drink (*action*) *juice* (*object*)
mummy (*agent*) *sing* (*action*)
eat (*action*) *dinner* (*object*)
daddy (*agent*) *dig* (*action*) *garden* (*object/location*)

5.3 Slang consists of highly informal, non-standard words and phrases that are usually avoided in formal speaking and writing. Jargon is the specialised vocabulary used by people in the same work or profession that allows members of that profession to communicate clearly and concisely with a minimum of ambiguity. Therefore, jargon will be used in formal speaking and writing.

6.1 the **tch** of *hutch* – voiceless post-alveolar affricate
the **c** of *cat* – voiceless velar plosive
the **ph** of *philosophy* – voiceless labio-dental fricative
the **se** of *nose* – voiced alveolar fricative
the **ng** of *wing* – voiced velar nasal
the **ll** of *yellow* – voiced alveolar lateral (approximant)
the **m** of *mouse* – voiced bilabial nasal

6.2 *plant* /plɑnt/   *mood* /mud/   *zebra* /zɛbrə/   *jaw* /dʒɔ/
bird /bɜd/   *nose* /nəʊz/   *thought* /θɔt/   *work* /wɜk/
talk /tɔk/   *ring* /rɪŋ/   *the* /ðə/   *red* /rɛd/
dent /dɛnt/   *fan* /fæn/   *shop* /ʃɒp/   *lamp* /læmp/
kiln /kɪln/   *vase* /vɑz/   *measure* /mɛʒə/   *yacht* /jɒt/
grow /grəʊ/   *sock* /sɒk/   *chop* /tʃɒp/   *house* /haʊs/

6.3 *pin*   /pɪn/   [pʰɪn]   *spin*   /spɪn/   [spɪ̃n]
pit   /pɪt/   [pʰɪtʰ]   *spit*   /spɪt/   [spɪtʰ]
Spain   /speɪn/   [speɪ̃n]   *map*   /mæp/   [mæ̃pʰ]

7.1 Phonemic, syllabic and word.

7.2 *flag* /flæg/ → [fæg] – initial cluster reduction
 snake /sneɪk/ → [səneɪk] – epenthesis
 police /pəˈlis/ → [ˈlis] – weak syllable deletion
 posts /pəʊsts/ → [pəʊs] – final cluster reduction
 case /keɪs/ → [seɪk] – metathesis
 cup /kʌp/ → [ʌp] – initial consonant deletion
 pat /pæt/ → [pæ] – final consonant deletion
 flow /fləʊ/ → [fəʊl] – metathesis
 bring /brɪŋ/ → [bərɪŋ] – epenthesis
 boat /bəʊt/ → [bəʊ] – final consonant deletion

7.3 *miss* /mɪs/ → [mɪt] – syllable-final stopping
 look /lʊk/ → [zʊk] – frication
 shed /ʃɛd/ → [fɛd] – syllable-initial palato-alveolar fronting
 door /dɔ/ → [gɔ] – syllable-initial backing
 love /lʌv/ → [jʌv] – gliding
 man /mæn/ → [bæn] – denasalisation
 pig /pɪg/ → [pɪd] – syllable-final velar fronting
 soap /səʊp/ → [təʊp] – syllable-initial stopping
 cart /kɑt/ → [tɑt] – syllable-initial velar fronting
 badge /bædʒ/ → [bæz] – syllable-final palato-alveolar fronting
 read /rid/ → [jid] – gliding
 hat /hæt/ → [hæk] – syllable-final backing
 ring /rɪŋ/ → [rɪg] – denasalisation

8.1 *this shoe* /ðɪs ʃu/ → [ðɪʃ ʃu]
 red pen /rɛd pɛn/ → [rɛb pɛn]
 matt black /mæt blæk/ → [mæp blæk]
 bad boy /bæd bɒɪ/ → [bæb bɒɪ]
 hit me /hɪt mi/ → [hɪp mi]
 seven pairs /sɛvən pɛəz/ → [sɛvəm pɛəz]
 his ship /hɪz ʃɪp/ → [hɪʒ ʃɪp]
 then make it /ðɛn meɪk ɪt/ → [ðɛm meɪk ɪt]

Miss Shepherd /mɪs ʃɛpəd/ → [mɪʃ ʃɛpəd]
those shells /ðəʊz ʃɛlz/ → [ðəʊʒ ʃɛlz]

8.2 *last time* /lɑst taɪm/ → [lɑs taɪm]
more of it /mɔ ɒv ɪt/ → [mɔr əv ɪt]
left bank /lɛft bæŋk/ → [lɛf bæŋk]
mashed potato /mæʃt pəteɪtəʊ/ → [mæʃ pəteɪtəʊ]
banned substance /bænd sʌbstəns/ → [bæn sʌbstəns]
here and now /hɪə ænd naʊ/ → [hɪər ən naʊ], [hɪər nd naʊ], etc.

8.3 Any two of: repetitions, prolongations, hesitations (blocks are typically only present in the speech of those who stammer).

9.1 Any three of: no predetermined cognitive map, collaboratively achieved, managed on a turn-by-turn basis, one-at-a-time talk, highly coordinated.

9.2 1   A   [TCU *he shows his fist to you does he?*] [TRP]
    2   B   [TCU *yeah*] [TRP] [TCU *he smoking all the time*] [TRP]
    3   A   [TCU *he's smoking all the time*] [TRP]
    4   B   [TCU *yeah*] [TRP]
    5   A   [TCU *yeah I know*] [TRP] [TCU *but tell him off*]

9.3 Extract A represents a violative interruption, as Lisa's line 2 talk commences on the second syllable of the word *pressing* uttered by Li Wei. This is not a valid transition relevance place. Extract B is an inadvertent overlap, as Sheilah commences her line 2 talk after the slight pause in Josie's utterance. This slight pause can be seen as signalling a transition relevance place. Josie had apparently not completed her turn at talk, however, as she tags on the phrase *or something like it*. Extract C is also an example of inadvertent overlap, as both Joe and Rob attempt to self-select themselves as next speaker under Rule 2. They do so at an appropriate transition relevance place that occurs at the end of Carl's line 1 turn-constructional unit.

Glossary

adjacency pair: a fundamental unit of conversation; sequences of two utterances that are adjacent, produced by different speakers, ordered as a first part and a second part, and typed so that a particular first part requires a particular second part.

adjective: a word that qualifies a noun or pronoun by providing additional and specific information (eg, *happy*, *tall*, *red*); a descriptor.

adverb: a word that is used to modify a verb, adjective or another adverb, typically providing circumstantial information such as the time, place, manner, degree or cause of an action or event (eg, *yesterday*, *outside*, *quickly*); may be temporal, locative, manner or intensifying.

affricate: a voiced or voiceless consonant constructed from a dynamic combination of complete closure within the oral cavity by the tongue contacting the alveolar ridge, followed immediately by near-closure and the consequent production of friction behind the alveolar ridge as the tongue moves backwards in the mouth.

agent: the animate (usually human) being who instigates a communicative behaviour by an act of will.

allophone: a phonetic variation of a phoneme that is insufficient to create a new word or meaning; its characteristics are typically influenced by its context of occurrence within a syllable.

approximant: a voiced consonant produced by near-closure within the oral cavity, but without friction being produced, ie, two articulators approximate closely together and the air is allowed to escape through the oral cavity in a continuous stream (sometimes known as *frictionless continuant*).

arbitrariness: a key property of language signifying that the choice of symbols used by a language is arbitrary, ie, there is no direct relationship between a particular word and its meaning.

articulators: structures within the vocal tract, such as the lips, teeth, tongue and palate, that are used to form speech sounds.

assimilation: the process whereby one speech segment is transposed into another owing to the influence of a neighbouring segment either within the same word or across a word boundary in connected speech, such as the dentalisation of alveolars when they occur in close proximity to dental fricatives, eg, *width* /wɪdθ/ → [wɪd̪θ].

babbling: the vocal play of babies at around six months of age, typified by stringing together sequences of consonants and vowels; may be reduplicated or non-reduplicated.

block: the coming together of two articulators with such excessive force that the speaker is unable to easily release the contact between them, resulting in a great deal of muscle tension; a principal indicator of stammering.

brain stem: upper extension of the spinal cord, situated beneath the cerebrum, that controls automatic functions such as heart rate and respiration, and reflex activities such as eye movement.

cerebellum: structure of the brain positioned towards the back of the skull, underneath the two cerebral hemispheres, that coordinates voluntary movements.

cerebrum: major structure of the brain that is divided along the longitudinal fissure into two almost identical halves – the left and right cerebral hemispheres; associated with reasoning ability, emotion, memory, motor movements, and speech and language skills.

clause: considered by some to be the largest syntactic unit, clauses are constructed of two or more phrases, one of which is always a verb phrase; there are seven clause structures in English – SVO, SV, SVA, SVC, SVOC, SVOA and SVOO.

cleft palate: a congenital anatomical impairment resulting from incomplete development of the tissues that form the soft palate, hard palate and lips; may result in articulation difficulties.

communication (human): an intentional act performed by a human agent for the purpose of causing some effect in an attentive human recipient.

competence: the ability to use an internalised grammar that enables one to both speak and understand an infinite number of potential utterances.

comprehension (see **receptive language**)

conjunction: a word that links other words, phrases and clauses (eg, *and*, *but*, *if*); may be coordinating or subordinating.

consonant: a closed speech sound produced by some type of obstruction to the airflow from the lungs by two articulators coming into contact with each other, or very nearly contacting, thus restricting the free flow of air.

conversation: the reciprocal, often informal, interactive discourse between two or more people; the archetypal language use through which people participate in social interactions.

cortex: the highly convoluted outer layer of the two cerebral hemispheres where intention, decision-making and thought arise.

cultural transmission: a key property of language signifying that language is the means by which humans are able to teach the upcoming generation all that they have learnt to date; communicating the necessary knowledge and social norms of behaviour to the upcoming generation through language.

determiner: a word occupying the first position in a noun phrase that determines what is being referred to by limiting the meaning of a noun (eg, *the*, *a*, *any*); may be an identifier or a quantifier.

diphthong: a complex vowel that involves two configurations of the oral cavity, ie, beginning with the articulation of one pure vowel the articulation is altered such that it moves smoothly towards the production of a second pure vowel.

displacement: a key property of language signifying that language allows us to think of, and communicate about, something or someone that is not immediately present, eg, as when we talk about our pet dog even though it is not present in the room with us.

duality: a key property of language signifying that language is organised at least at two levels, with the elements of the secondary level (speech sounds) combining to form the units of the primary level (words).

elision: the deletion of a sound, or sounds, either within a word or across a word boundary in connected speech, eg, *best day* /bɛst deɪ/ → [bɛs deɪ].

expressive language: the ability to encode and produce meaningful utterances through an appropriate use of vocabulary, syntax and morphology.

fluency: the smooth, uninterrupted flow of speech.

fricative: a voiced or voiceless consonant produced by air from the lungs forcing its way through a narrow gap created in the oral cavity by two articulators coming into near contact, such that friction or turbulence is created.

genderlect: an aspect of language use that marks asymmetry in power relationships, real or imagined, between men and women; most often disparaging of the female gender.

grammar: the set of rules that governs how the various symbols of language (words) may be combined to form meaningful utterances.

hearing: the physiological and anatomical capacity to detect (speech) sounds.

hesitation: a halt in the free flow of speech; may be silent or filled pauses.

holophrase: single words used by infants, usually up to the age of 2;00 years, that have the force of a whole phrase which would normally be made up of several adult words.

inadvertent overlap: when the talk of two or more participants in a conversation accidentally overlaps at a potential transition relevance place.

language: the ability to understand and use verbal symbols; the predominant means by which human beings communicate with each other.

language acquisition device (LAD): a term proposed by the linguist Noam Chomsky to refer to a child's innate general language-learning ability; the blueprint in the brain that allows a child to recognise the structure-dependence of language and to manipulate these structures.

larynx: anatomical cartilaginous structure at the upper end of the trachea that contains the vocal folds.

liaison: the process operating in connected speech whereby a vowel in word-final position is linked by the insertion of an /r/ sound to an immediately following vowel in word-initial position, eg, *more over* /mɔ əʊvə/ → [mɔɹ əʊvə].

linguistic development: the stage of development, from around 1;00 to 5;00 years of age, when children develop the capacity to understand and use verbal symbols; divided into six stages – Early One Word, Later One Word, Two Word, Three Word, Four Word and Complex Utterance.

linguistics: the scientific study of language.

listening: the active attention to (speech) sounds.

monophthong: a simple, or pure vowel, produced by assuming only a single configuration of the oral cavity, ie, there is no movement of the tongue, lips or jaws during production.

morpheme: the smallest element in a language capable of creating a distinction in meaning; root, prefix or suffix.

morphology: the study of word formation in a particular language, focusing especially on the internal structure of the words and their alteration through the addition of prefixes and suffixes.

motherese: the (unconscious) modifications of a caregiver's expressive language when speaking to an infant, thought to assist the child with language-learning, eg, speaking in monologues, restricting the number of topics, repetition of words and phrases.

nasal: a voiced consonant sound produced by a complete obstruction in the oral cavity, by the lips coming together or the tongue contacting the alveolar ridge or velum, and with the soft palate lowered so that the air escapes in a continuous stream through the nasal cavity.

non-verbal communication: the variety of ways, systematic and non-systematic, in which human beings transmit meaning to one another other than by spoken language (sometimes known as *non-oral communication*).

noun: a word used to name a person, place, thing, action, and so on (eg, *Margaret, Billingham, book, (a) shot*); may be proper, common, concrete, abstract, countable or mass.

numeral: a word that expresses a number or the sequential order of something (eg, *one, five, third*); may be cardinal or ordinal.

orthography: a method of writing text using a fixed number of symbols (alphabetic letters) that do not necessarily bear a one-to-one relationship to the sounds of a particular language.

over-extension: common up to about 2;00 years of age, the use of the same word to refer to many different things, eg, when the word *dog* is used to mean all animals, whether or not the animal being referred to is a cat, a horse, a pig, or whatever.

performance: the behaviour of producing actual utterances that may or may not be perceived as grammatically correct.

phoneme: the smallest element of speech capable of creating a distinction in meaning between different spoken words.

phonemic transcription: a method of representing speech sounds in written form such that each symbol used represents only one speech sound.

phonetics: the aspect of the study of speech that describes how the various speech sounds are articulated and combined.

phonological simplifying process: the simplification of the pronunciation of a phonological unit through either structural alterations, such as consonant deletion and cluster reduction, or systemic changes, such as the systematic substitution of sounds or the assimilation of one sound to another.

phonology: the study of the rule system that governs how particular speech sounds are used to produce meaningful words; the systematic organisation of sounds in a particular language.

phrase: a syntactic unit at an intermediate level of organisation between the word and the clause, typically constructed of a sequence of two or more words; may be a verb phrase, noun phrase, adverb phrase, adjective phrase or prepositional phrase.

pitch: the human perception of how high or low the note produced by the vibration of the vocal folds appears to be; related to the frequency of vibration of the vocal folds.

plosive: an oral voiced or voiceless consonant produced by a complete obstruction of the airflow from the lungs, by the lips coming together or the tongue contacting the alveolar ridge or velum, followed by the explosive release of the air through the mouth as the two articulators part suddenly.

pragmatics: the study of the use of language in its social context; the study of meaning derived from context.

pre-linguistic development: the stage of development, from birth to around 1;01 years of age, prior to the child being able to understand and use verbal symbols; divided into four stages – reflexive crying and vegetative sounds, cooing and laughter, vocal play and babbling.

preposition: a word placed before a noun phrase to indicate its relationship to a verb, adjective, noun or pronoun (eg, *in*, *of*, *for*).

productivity: a key property of language signifying that language can be used to construct an infinite set of new and meaningful utterances that are readily interpretable by other people.

prolongation: a lengthening of the normal duration of vowels and continuant consonants; rare in normal speech, but common in stammering.

pronoun: a word that substitutes for a noun (eg, *I*, *it*, *she*); may be personal, reflexive, demonstrative, interrogative or indefinite.

prosody: features of connected speech such as rhythm and intonation, the effects of which go beyond single segments and affect the whole utterance, being simultaneously compiled with the segmental features (speech sounds, syllables, words, phrases); the characteristic rhythmical beat of connected speech and its attendant musical quality.

receptive language: the ability to decode and understand verbal symbols.

repetition: a repeating of speech sounds, syllables, words or phrases in connected speech; often the first sign of stammering.

schwa: the simple vowel /ə/ that is made with spread lips and the tongue held mid-way between a high and low position in the mouth; only occurs in unstressed syllables; sometimes known as the neutral vowel.

semantic category: a category of meaning, grouping together words that appear to perform the same semantic function in an utterance, eg, *mummy* and *daddy* may function as AGENT, *house* and *garden* may function as LOCATION, *kick* and *sing* may function as ACTION.

semantics: the study of the meaning of linguistic tokens such as words, phrases and clauses; the study of which tokens are used, how they make reference to things, ideas, emotions, etc, and how the hearer interprets them.

sentence: a syntactic unit, usually consisting of more than one clause, that appears to convey a complete thought.

specialisation: a key property of language signifying that language allows us to substitute an arbitrary word for a physical action, eg, a police officer who instructs a person to 'Move along!' has used language to substitute for the physical action of physically pushing the person forwards.

speech: the complex learned transmission system of language which involves the coordinated use of voice and articulation to produce sounds that are used to form meaningful words.

stammer: disruption of the free flow of speech owing to excessive, unplanned repetitions, prolongations, hesitations and blocks (sometimes known as *stutter*).

structural simplification: a phonological simplifying process that involves some alteration to the internal structure of a particular word, such as the deletion of consonants and the reduction of consonant clusters.

structure-dependence: a key property of language signifying the underlying patterned structure of language, ie, language naturally patterns into the building blocks of phrases which may be variously rearranged and substituted.

style shifting: the (often intentional) alteration of morphology, syntax, vocabulary and phonology to produce either a more formal, prescriptive utterance or a less formal, functional utterance that reflects a particular dialect and/or accent.

syllable: a unit of spoken language that is constructed from phonemes and uttered as an unbroken sound; an intermediate level of phonological organisation between the phoneme and the word.

syntax: the rules that govern the combination of words and their sequential placement, in order to create meaningful grammatical phrases and clauses.

systematicity: a key property of language signifying that the production of language is not a random act, but that specific rules are followed that govern how elements at both the secondary level and units at the primary level are combined, eg, /k/, /æ/ and /t/ combine to form the primary level unit *cat* /kæt/, but not *atc* /ætk/.

systemic simplification: a phonological simplifying process that involves the systematic variation of a particular type of speech sound and its replacement with another speech sound, eg, when alveolar sounds are systematically substituted by sounds made at the back of the mouth or when fricative sounds are stopped.

transition relevance place: the end of a turn-constructional unit in a conversation where the participants may alternate, ie, the current speaker becomes the current listener and the current listener becomes the current speaker.

turn-constructional unit: the various utterances that the current speaker in a conversation makes; syntactic units like noun phrase, verb phrase, and so on, readily identifiable by prosodic features such as pitch-height, tempo and loudness variations.

under-extension: common up to about 2;00 years of age, the restricted use of a single word that could appropriately be applied to many objects, people, etc, to only one or two things, eg, when the word *drink* is used to refer solely to orange squash and not to any other drink.

verb: a word that expresses an action, a state of being or an event (eg, *running, presume, arrived*); may be auxiliary or lexical.

violative interruption: a transgression of the rules of turn-allocation by a participant in a conversation who wilfully interrupts the current speaker by talking when there is no viable transition relevance place.

vocabulary: all the words of a particular world language; the sum of all the words used by a person or group of people.

vocal apparatus: the anatomical structures used to produce speech sounds, consisting of the breathing mechanism, the larynx, and the vocal tract.

vocal tract: the air passages above the larynx, consisting of the nasal and oral cavities.

voice: the sound produced in the larynx by the vibration of the two vocal folds.

voiced: label used to describe the voicing of a speech sound, ie, if the sound (vowel or consonant) is produced with the vocal folds vibrating then the speech sound is voiced.

voiceless: label used to describe the voicing of a speech sound, ie, if the sound (consonant) is produced without the vocal folds vibrating then the speech sound is voiceless.

volume: the human perception of how loud or soft the sound produced by the vibration of the vocal folds appears to be; related to the intensity of the vibration of the vocal folds.

vowel: an open speech sound that involves no obstruction to the airflow from the lungs; may be simple (monophthong) or complex (diphthong).

vowel reduction: the process whereby the strong form of a vowel is reduced to a weak form in connected speech, eg, *of* /ɒv/ reducing to the weak form [əv] in the phrase *man of means*.

word: a unit of meaning in a language, consisting minimally of one morpheme (root) that may be expanded by the addition of prefixes and suffixes; a unit of meaning in spoken language that represents the highest level of phonological organisation, being composed of syllables that are themselves composed of phonemes; may be monosyllabic or polysyllabic.

Bibliography

Aitchison J, 1976, *The Articulate Mammal*, Hutchinson, London.

Ayto J (ed), 1999, *The Oxford Dictionary of Slang*, Oxford Paperbacks, Oxford.

Berko J, 1958, 'The Child's Learning of English Morphology', *Word* 14, pp150–77.

Blom L, 1973, *One Word at a Time*, Mouton, The Hague.

Bloom L, (ed), 1993, *Language Development from Two to Three*, Cambridge University Press, Cambridge.

Brown R, 1958, *Words and Things*, The Free Press, New York.

Brown R, 1973, *A First Language*, Allen & Unwin, London.

Burke P & Porter R, 1995, *Languages and Jargons: Contributions to a Social History of Language*, Polity Press, Oxford.

Chomsky N, 1965, *Aspects of the Theory of Syntax*, MIT Press, Cambridge, Mass.

Chomsky N, 1972, *Language and Mind*, Harcourt Brace Jovanovich, New York.

Clark J & Yallop C, 1995, *An Introduction to Phonetics and Phonology*, 2nd edn, Blackwell, Oxford.

Coates J, 1993, *Women, Men and Language*, 2nd edn, Longman, London.

Crystal D, 1986, *Listen to Your Child*, Penguin, Harmondsworth.

Crystal D & Varley R, 1998, *Introduction to Language Pathology*, 4th edn, Whurr Publishers, London.

Curtis S, Fromkin V, Krashen D, Rigler D & Rigler M, 1974, 'The Linguistic Development of Genie', *Language* 50, pp528–54.

Denes PB & Pinson EN, 1973, *The Speech Chain*, Anchor Press, New York.

Denes PB & Pinson EN, 1993, *The Speech Chain*, WH Freeman, Basingstoke.

Dore J, 1975, 'Holophrases, Speech Acts, and Language Universals', *Journal of Child Language* 2, pp21–40.

Drach K, 1969, 'The Language of the Parent: A Pilot Study', *Working Paper Number 4: The Structure of Linguistic Input to Children*, University of California Language Behavior Research Laboratory, Berkeley.

Edelsky C, 1981, 'Who's Got the Floor?', *Language in Society* 10, pp383–421.

Ervin-Tripp S, 1964, 'Imitation and Structural Change in Children's Language', Lenneberg EH (ed), *New Directions in the Study of Language*, MIT Press, Cambridge,

Mass.

Gannon PJ, Holloway RL, Broadfield DC & Braun AR, 1998, 'Asymmetry of Chimpanzee Planum Temporale: Humanlike Pattern of Wernicke's Brain Language Area Homolog', *Science* 279, pp220–22.

Gardner RA & Gardner BT, 1969, 'Teaching Sign Language to a Chimpanzee', *Science* 165, pp664–72.

Gardner RA & Gardner BT, 1989, 'A Cross-Fostering Laboratory', Gardner RA, Gardner BT & Van Cantfort TE (eds), *Teaching Sign Language to Chimpanzees*, State University of New York Press, New York.

Gregory H, 1999, *Semantics: An Introductory Workbook*, Routledge, London.

Griffin E, 1996, *A First Look at Communication Theory*, 3rd edn, McGraw-Hill Publishing, New York.

Halliday MAK, 1975, *Learning How to Mean: Explorations in the Development of Language*, Edward Arnold, London.

Hardcastle WJ & Hewlett N (eds), 1999, *Coarticulation: Theory, Data and Techniques in Speech Production*, Cambridge University Press, Cambridge.

Harris J, 1990, *Early Language Development: Implications for Educational and Clinical Practice*, Routledge, London.

Hockett CF, 1963, 'The Problem of Universals in Language', Greenberg JH (ed), *Universals of Language*, MIT Press, Cambridge, Mass.

Hudson RA, 1996, *Sociolinguistics*, 2nd edn, Cambridge University Press, Cambridge.

International Phonetic Association, 1999, *Handbook of the International Phonetic Association*, Cambridge University Press, Cambridge.

IUPAC, 1993, *A Guide to IUPAC Nomenclature of Organic Compounds (Recommendations 1993)*, Blackwell Scientific, Oxford.

Jackson H, 1990, *Grammar and Meaning: A Semantic Approach to English Grammar*, Longman, Harlow.

James E, 1999, *Contemporary British Slang*, National Textbook Company, Lincolnwood, IL.

Kellogg WN & Kellogg LA, 1933, *The Ape and the Child*, McGraw Hill, New York.

Klima E & Bellugi U, 1966, 'Syntactic Regularities in the Speech of Children', Lyons J & Wales RJ (eds), *Psycholinguistic Papers*, Edinburgh University Press, Edinburgh.

Knowles W & Masidlover M, 1982, *Derbyshire Language Scheme*, Derbyshire County Council, Derby.

Lenneberg EH, 1967, *Biological Foundations of Language*, Wiley, New York.

Levinson SC, 1983, *Pragmatics*, Cambridge University Press, Cambridge.

Linden E, 1974, *Apes, Men and Language*, Saturday Review Press, New York.

Local J, Kelly J & Wells WHG, 1986, 'Towards a Phonology of Conversation: Turn-Taking in Tyneside English', *Journal of Linguistics,* 22, pp411–38.

Martin S, 1987, *Working with Dysphonics*, Winslow Press, Bicester.

Martini F & Welch K, 1999, *Fundamentals of Anatomy and Physiology*, 4th edn, Prentice Hall, Englewood Cliffs, NJ.

McTear M, 1985, *Children's Conversation*, Blackwell, Oxford.

Miles HLW, 1993, 'Language and the Orang-utan: The Old "Person" of the Forest',

Cavalieri P & Singer P (eds), *The Great Ape Project: Equality Beyond Humanity*, St Martin's Press, New York.

Miller JF, 1981, 'Eliciting Procedures for Language', Miller JF (ed), *Assessing Language Production in Children*, Edward Arnold, London.

Piaget J, 1952, *The Origins of Intelligence in Children*, International Universities Press, New York.

Premack AJ, 1976, *Why Chimps Can Read*, Harper & Row, New York.

Premack D, 1970, 'The Education of Sarah', *Psychology Today*, 4, pp55–58.

Premack D, 1971, 'Language in Chimpanzee?', *Science*, 172, pp808–22.

Quirk R & Greenbaum S, 1973, *A Concise Grammar of Contemporary English*, Harcourt Brace Jovanovich, New York.

Reisman K, 1974, 'Contrapuntal Conversations in an Antiguan Village', Bauman R & Sherzer J (eds), *Explorations in the Ethnography of Speaking*, Cambridge University Press, Cambridge.

Ringler NM, 1981, 'The Development of Language and How Adults Talk to Children', *Infant Mental Health*, 2, pp71–83.

Sacks H, Schegloff EA & Jefferson G, 1974, 'A Simplest Systematics for the Organization of Turn-Taking in Conversation', *Language*, 50, 4, pp696–735. (*Variant version published as Sacks, Schegloff & Jefferson, 1978*)

Sacks H, Schegloff EA & Jefferson G, 1978, 'A Simplest Systematics for the Organization of Turn-Taking in Conversation', Schenkein J (ed), *Studies in the Organization of Conversational Interaction*, Academic Press, New York.

Savage-Rumbaugh S & Lewin R, 1994, *Kanzi: The Ape at the Brink of the Human Mind*, John Wiley & Sons, New York.

Schegloff EA & Sacks H, 1973, 'Opening up Closings', *Semiotica* 7, 4, pp289–327.

Schiffrin D, 1994, *Approaches to Discourse*, Blackwell, Oxford.

Skinner BF, 1957, *Verbal Behavior*, Appleton-Century-Crofts, New York.

Slobin D, 1967, *A Field Manual for Cross-Cultural Study of the Acquisition of Communicative Competence*, University of California, Berkeley.

Smith N & Wilson D, 1979, *Modern Linguistics: The Result of Chomsky's Revolution*, Penguin Books, London.

Stark RE, 1986, 'Prespeech Segmental Feature Development', Fletcher P & Garman M (eds), *Language Acquisition*, 2nd edn, Cambridge University Press, Cambridge.

Terrace HS, 1979, *Nim*, Alfred A Knopf, New York.

Verschueren J, 1998, *Understanding Pragmatics*, Arnold, London.

Wallman J, 1992, *Aping Language*, Cambridge University Press, Cambridge.

Williamson G, 1995, *Instructor-Trainee Conversation in an Adult Training Centre for People with Learning Disabilities: An Analysis of the Function and Distribution of Back Channel Tokens and Personal Names*, unpublished PhD thesis, University of Newcastle upon Tyne, Newcastle.

Further Reading

This is a guide to basic texts for the reader who is new to the subject of human communication. Further references can be obtained by consulting these recommended texts.

Chapter 1: The Nature of Human Communication

Cook VJ, 1997, *Inside Language*, Arnold, London.
Deacon T, 1998, *The Symbolic Species: The Co-Evolution of Language and the Human Brain*, Penguin Books, London.
Pinker S, 2000, *The Language Instinct: The New Science of Language and Mind*, Penguin Books, London.
Ruben BD, Stewart LP & Stewart L, 1998, *Communication & Human Behavior*, 4th edn, Allyn & Bacon, Needham Heights, Mass.

Chapter 2: Language Properties, Acquisition and Development

Aitchison J, 1996, *The Language Web: The Power and Problem of Words – the 1996 BBC Reith Lectures*, Cambridge University Press, Cambridge.
Cattell R, 2000, *Children's Language: Consensus and Controversy*, Continuum Publishing Group, London.
Myszor F, 1999, *Language Acquisition*, Hodder & Stoughton Educational, London.
Savage-Rumbaugh ES, Shanker S & Taylor TJ, 1998, *Apes, Language and the Human Mind*, Oxford University Press Inc, New York.
Trask RL (ed), 1997, *A Student's Dictionary of Language and Linguistics*, Arnold, London.

Chapters 3–4: Grammar, Morphology and Syntax

Graddol D, Cheshire J & Swann J, 1994, *Describing Language*, 2nd edn, Open University Press, Milton Keynes.

Greenbaum S, 1991, *An Introduction to English Grammar*, Longman Higher Education, Harlow.
Leech G, 1990, *An A–Z of English Grammar and Usage*, Longman ELT, London.
Shiach D, 1995, *Basic Grammar*, John Murray, London.

Chapter 5: Semantics, Pragmatics and Sociolinguistics

Chierchia G & McConnell-Ginet S, 2000, *Meaning and Grammar: An Introduction to Semantics*, 2nd edn, MIT Press, Cambridge, Mass.
Cruse A, 1999, *Meaning in Language: An Introduction to Semantics and Pragmatics*, Oxford University Press, Oxford.
Dunbar R, 1997, *Grooming, Gossip and the Evolution of Language*, Faber & Faber, London.
Holmes J, 1992, *An Introduction to Sociolinguistics*, Longman Higher Education, Harlow.
Mey JL, 1993, *Pragmatics: An Introduction*, Blackwell Publishers, Oxford.
Peccei JS, 1999, *Pragmatics*, Routledge, London.
Trudgill P, 1995, *Sociolinguistics: An Introduction to Language and Society*, Penguin Books, London.

Chapters 6–8: Phonetics and Phonology

Bloodstein O, 1995, *Handbook on Stuttering*, 5th edn, Singular Press, California.
Couper-Kuhlen E & Selting M (eds), 1996, *Prosody in Conversation: Interactional Studies*, Cambridge University Press, Cambridge.
Davenport M & Hannahs SJ, 1998, *Introducing Phonetics and Phonology*, Arnold, London.
House L, 1998, *Introductory Phonetics and Phonology: A Workbook Approach*, Lawrence Erlbaum Associates, Mahwah, NJ.
Ladefoged P, 1993, *A Course in Phonetics*, 3rd edn, Harcourt Publishers School Department, Philadelphia.
Roach P, 1991, *English Phonetics and Phonology: a Practical Course*, 2nd edn, Cambridge University Press, Cambridge.
Trask RL, 1995, *A Dictionary of Phonetics and Phonology*, Routledge, London.

Chapter 9: Conversation

Eggins S & Slade D, 1997, *Analysing Casual Conversations*, Continuum Publishing Group, London.
ten Have P, 1998, *Doing Conversation Analysis: A Practical Guide*, Sage Publications Ltd, London.
Wooffitt R & Hutchby I, 1998, *Conversation Analysis: Principles, Practices and Applications*, Polity Press, Oxford.
Zeldin T, 1998, *Conversation*, Harvill Press, London.

Index

INDEX